STOP DRINKING
ALCOHOL

**Complete Cure Guide To Overcome
Alcoholism: Sobriety In 30 Days. The
Effective Way To Recover From Alcohol
Addiction, Be Free And Quit Drinking.**

DWIGHT HORTON

Table of Contents

INTRODUCTION

Alcohol is a very ancient drink that has been consumed for thousands of years by almost all civilizations. Alcoholic beverages are an important part of many social events. A lot of us resort to a glass of wine at home after a hard day. So how do you know when an innocent drink turns into a dangerous addiction? Can alcohol actually be good for you? What is a safe dose of alcohol? We set out on a quest to find out the answers to all these questions and more.

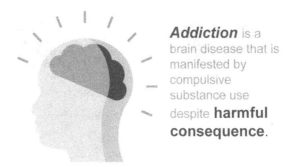

Addiction is a brain disease that is manifested by compulsive substance use despite **harmful consequence**.

So can alcohol actually be used as a medicine? The answer is only in rare cases. If we are dealing with a heart attack, liver or kidney colic and there are no medications available, then we can use alcohol. One tablespoon of vodka or cognac will help eliminate the vessel and muscular spasms thus improving the patient's condition until the ambulance arrives. However the relaxation effect caused by alcohol is very short and is followed by the phase of prolonged vessel and muscular spasms.

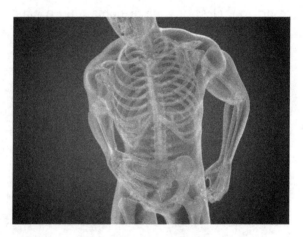

What effects do alcoholic beverages have on blood pressure? They raise it. This is exactly the reason why alcohol actually helps those who have hypotonia, one or two tablespoons of cognac can resuscitate a person with low blood pressure. However, the World Health Organization does not recommend for doctors to advise their patients to take any alcoholic beverages as their medicine. Longstanding research shows that the cause of 20% of all cases of hypertension is alcohol, especially beer and vodka. Thus, if a man consumes more than 5 oz of wine or 2 oz of vodka a day, the risk of developing hypertension increases to 40%; in the same case for women the risk increases to 90%! So it is much safer to increase blood pressure not with alcohol but with coffee, tea, dark chocolate, or ginseng tincture.

It's a known fact that natural dry wines are beneficial for us. What is this effect due to? The skin and seeds of red type of grape contain a substance that has a huge antioxidant effect. When we eat that type of grapes or drink wine made out of it, this substance prevents the development of cardio-vascular and oncological diseases, it slows down the age changes in the brain and in the motor function thus extending the life span and delaying the body's aging. Besides that, alcoholic beverages improve digestion and prevent building up of cholesterol on the vascular walls. But all of this is true only when alcohol is consumed in moderate amounts. Consumption of alcohol in large amounts leads to heart pathologies and hypertension. So it's much safer to lower cholesterol with the help of physical activities and rational diet, which are just as effective as alcohol.

How is it that the French eat a lot of fatty foods, drink beer and at the same time live long lives and suffer from cardio-vascular diseases 40% less than the Americans? The secret of the "French paradox" is not only in consuming wine regularly, but also in their lifestyle and peculiarities of their diet. Besides wine and cheese the French consume a large amount of vegetables, fruit, verdure, olive oil and seafood. This diet supplies the body with lipoproteins of high density, unsaturated fats, vitamins and microelements, which cause a powerful antioxidant effect, protecting the body's cells from damages by free radicals. Furthermore, the residents of South France actively consume seaweed, which contains substances that improve the biological properties of blood (decrease the formation of clots and stimulate disintegration of fats).

What amount of alcohol is considered a safe dose? In France, Italy, and Hungary this number would traditionally be higher than that in Sweden or Norway, for example. But talking about the common dose, the World Health Organization recommends for men to consume not more than 30 ml of pure alcohol, which is about 1.5 bottles of beer or 2 shots of vodka a day, and for women - 20 ml of pure alcohol per day, which is 1 bottle of beer or 1 shot of vodka. The doctors also recommend refraining from drinking alcoholic beverages at least two days a week.

So why is the safe dose for women lower than the one for men? This is explained by the fact that women have less water in their body than men do. Besides, the element responsible for the disintegration of alcohol located in the stomach is less active in women. Therefore the processing of alcoholic beverages is slower in female bodies making the ladies more receptive to alcohol.

Why is it that some people get a headache after a glass of red wine, but feel fine after drinking white wine? This reaction could be caused by individual intolerance of sulfur dioxide - the substance that is added to red dry wines for longer storage. This preservative can cause immediate redness of the face and strong migraines. This does not happen when consuming white wines because there is no sulfur dioxide added to them according to their preparation technology.

How safe are the low-alcohol sparkling drinks so popular among the younger people? Easy math allows us to see that this category of drinks is not so harmless. Most of them contain 8% alcohol. If you multiply this number by 0.33, which is the contents of one bottle, then we get about 27 ml of pure alcohol. For women it is already over their daily limit, and usually few stop at just one bottle a day. Besides these drinks usually contain carbon dioxide, which contributes to faster absorption of alcohol into blood due to which intoxication happens almost after the first sip.

What are the consequences of immoderate consumption of beer? Beer, just as any other alcoholic beverage, first of all affects the liver, causing toxic hepatitis and alcohol cirrhosis. Namely these two diseases have the leading positions in beer countries such as Germany, where beer is consumed often and in big amounts, up to 3 liters per night.

Former smokers complain that after having a drink they get the desire to smoke again. Why does it happen? Usually this happens to those who managed to say no to the harmful habit but haven't coped with the psychological smoking addiction. Once the former smoker goes to the party where a lot of people smoke, he or she can experience what a former drug addict would feel if he appeared in a surrounding where they used to do drugs. Just one glance at the familiar surroundings is enough to be overtaken with the associative habit. Under the influence of alcohol, the memory draws the pictures of the past that are so vivid that the former smoker can actually feel the taste and smell of tobacco. Besides being in the state of euphoria (after having a couple of drinks) a person already can not critically assess his or her actions and breaks their own promises without thinking twice. Typically we smoke more cigarettes than usual in this condition. As a result the toxic effect of alcohol is intensified by several times, hence a more severe hangover.

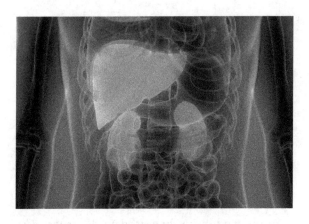

What medicines could be combined with alcohol? Alcohol is not compatible with any medications, especially cardio-stimulants, tranquilizers, antidepressants, and beta-blockers. Losing conciseness is the least of the potential consequences. Sometimes alcohol can intensify the effects of the medications by so much that it can lead to coma or even sudden death. Alcoholic beverages are also not compatible with diuretic medications. Combined with wine or beer diuretics remove such a big amount of microelements out of your body that it can lead to heart malfunctions. Even the commonplace aspirin should not be chased with alcoholic drinks - such experiments can lead to stomach ulcer. A vast amount of complications can be caused by combining alcohol with antibiotics. Not all medications enter our body in active form. A lot of them start acting only after they pass the stage of disintegration in the liver. Alcohol requires disintegration too, and thus once both medications and alcohol enter our body at the same time, both of these substances start to compete. As a result the active ingredient of the medication gets to our body under-oxidized, which most often leads to allergic reactions.

Why is it that some people become placid and talkative after having a drink, and others become withdrawn and aggressive? In spite of the person's character, age and mood, the alcohol slows down the function of the nervous system. Two minutes after having a drink, the alcohol reaches the frontal lobe of the brain leading to the disruption of the most of neuro-chemical bonds. You become absent-minded, the thoughts become chaotic, and the mood becomes elevated and cheerful. Although this state of euphoria is short-term, soon the phase of inhibition comes, during which the intoxicated person looses restraint and common sense and their conversations and actions become inappropriate. Usually alcohol affects healthy people as an emotional equalizer: a closed-off person brightens up after a glass of wine, a talkative one quiets down, an aggressive one calms down. Although sometimes unexpected reactions happen, which are usually predetermined by peculiarities of the person's nervous system. One fact remains though, if after having a drink you become aggressive, you should stay away from drinking.

A lot of people consider alcohol the best cure of stress, is that true? Alcohol is the most simple and accessible tranquilizer. However it does not relieve stress, otherwise everyone would be drinking their problems away. Fortunately, this does not happen since for most people alcohol is just a mediator, something of a relaxing element, which allows them to talk frankly, to pour their heart out to the closest friend, neighbor, and fellow traveler. However the doctors consider jogging just as effective due to the increased production of energy in our body when under stress. That is why when we start stressing out we cannot stay in one place: we pace the room, pull at our hair, talk emotionally. Therefore it would be quite logical to get rid of the excess energy at the gym rather than at the bar.

Are there any rules one should follow when drinking? The first rule is never drink on an empty stomach. If you don't eat anything prior, alcohol is absorbed freely by the stomach and quickly gets into blood causing immediate and very strong intoxication. This is why dietitians recommend eating something greasy beforehand. The second rule is to start the party up with aperitif, a small drink before you eat to stimulate the appetite. If you have a little bit of wine, vodka or martini first, not only will you stimulate the appetite, but you will also make the fermentative system work more actively. The third rule is if you have to change a drink make sure to drink higher proof drinks each time. Processing high-proof drinks requires a lot of the ferment responsible for breaking up alcohol hence if you chase cognac with champagne you will cause the deficit of this ferment. Because of that, the low-proof drink gets into our body unbroken without obstruction causing strong intoxication.

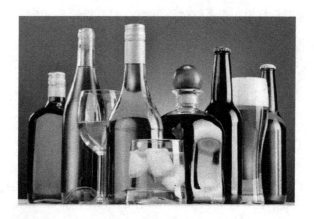

What kind of food should you have with strong drinks? Dry wines should be followed by fruit, cheese, salads, non-greasy types of meat, and fish. Drinks with 80 proof and higher go best with greasier and heavier foods - pork, lamb, red caviar, potatoes, salads with high-calories sauces. This will help slow down the absorption of alcohol and improve the digestion of food since alcohol helps break up fats. It is desirable to have fresh lemons available during a long get-together. The acid contained by them is an excellent decomposer of alcohol therefore you can chase your drinks with cut up pieces of this sour fruit or have a glass of water mixed with lemon juice. You might want to get rid of sparkling sweet drinks since sugar and carbon dioxide contained by them increase the absorption speed of alcohol. This is the same reason why you should not chase sparkling wines with chocolate.

What is alcohol poisoning? What are its symptoms and what precautions should be taken to save the person who got alcohol poisoning? Alcohol poisoning happens after consumption of more than 500 ml of vodka. Most people's body natural reaction to such an amount of toxic substances is vomiting, but more than 30% of alcohol drinkers are missing this reflex, therefore if the body is exposed to a large amount of ethanol, it undergoes the strongest alcohol intoxication: alcohol paralyzes the nervous system which leads to comatose condition and if left unattended can lead to death in several hours. This is why if you find someone unconscious with a distinct alcohol smell, pale, perspirating, having hurried breathing, not reacting to any outside stimuli, having weak pulse and uneven heartbeat, call the ambulance immediately.

DEFINITION OF ALCOHOLISM

There are many definitions of alcoholism. The most common definition of alcoholism is that "alcoholism is a horrible disease that affects the whole person ". However this definition may also apply to cancer or other dreadful diseases. Alcoholism cannot be defined simply as a disease caused by prolonged consumption of alcohol. The amount and frequency of drinking will determine alcoholism.

A more accurate definition of alcoholism suggests a chronic disorder characterized by some loss of control over drinking. Drinking more frequently and at inappropriate times will point towards alcoholism. Alcoholism is a common term for two distinct disorders. They are alcohol abuse and alcohol dependence.

The medical definition of alcoholism describes alcoholism as a disease caused by continuous consumption of alcohol. The quantity and frequency of alcohol consumption required to develop alcoholism will vary from person to person.

Alcoholism is also qualified by some other expressions. They include use, misuse, heavy use, abuse and dependence. Use is a term which simply refers to a person who drinks any alcoholic products. Misuse and heavy use do not have any standard definitions. Heavy use of alcohol will vary from person to person depending upon the age, alcohol brand and so on.

Alcohol abuse is one of the serious problems which lead to poor nutrition, memory loss, difficulty in walking and liver diseases. It will also generate mental stress, depression, fatigue, employment problems, family problems etc. Alcohol abuse may also involve the drinker in legal problems at some point in his life. The drinker will continue to drink at this stage irrespective of his health and family problems.

Addiction to alcohol will cause alcohol dependency. Alcohol dependence will cause social and work related problems. The drinker will experience periods of shaking, sweating and nausea when he tries to stop drinking when he reaches the stage of addiction. Alcohol dependence is usually indicated if the following symptoms are present:

1. Increases in level of tolerance to alcohol.

2. The drinker will take more alcohol to avoid withdrawal symptoms.

3. He will lose control over drinking.

4. He may spend more time in drinking and will recover from it only after long period of time.

5. He will lose interest in social and recreational activities.

6. He will continue to drink though he knows the adverse effects of drinking.

Alcoholism will lead most of the alcoholics to increase their consumption. Loss of control will happen in this stage. In fact loss of control is a clear symptom of alcoholism. As the drinker continues to drink, his body will build increased tolerance towards alcohol. Therefore the drinker will not get fully content by consuming the usual amount of alcohol. He will need more and more. Withdrawal symptoms like nausea, sweating and shaking will also appear.

Alcohol problems will vary from person to person. The severity of alcoholism will also vary from drinker to drinker. Some may experience life threatening problems. Liver dysfunction, brain disorders etc will also occur. Rightly said, alcoholism is a horrible disease. However it is possible to cure the disease. Alcoholics Anonymous have helped millions through their method of sharing their experiences amongst themselves as long as the member desires to stop drinking. Health Coaching is another method in which the alcoholic recognizes the effects of his behavior on his body, his family and his surroundings and obtains personalized help to take action and continue his sobriety.

DEFINITION OF ALCOHOLISM - RELEVANT OR NOT?

With many different opinions and approaches it is not easy to give a definition of alcoholism. Definitions in general often evoke contrasting views which can be rather confusing. In America alcoholism is accepted as a disease, whereas in Europe generally, it is not seen as a medical problem, and therefore hardly any funds are made available to find a 'medical solution'.

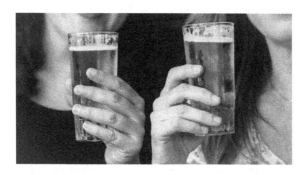

The definition of alcoholism remains vague but overall we can say that alcoholism is a form of problem drinking and involves a physical dependence on alcoholic drinks.

But what about the people affected by it? Are they interested in a fancy definition? Probably not. Partners, family members and friends of alcoholics are trying to make sense of a life out of control, a life of lies. People are trying to make ends meet and there is desperation and often violence, both verbally and physically. They don't care about fancy studies and conclusions and are more interested in advice on living with an alcoholic and how to help an alcoholic.

The alcoholic, held hostage by the alcohol, feels alone and in deep conflict with those around him and deep down inside, also with him or herself. They probably know the problems alcohol abuse can cause. They probably know what it must mean to their loved ones to live with an alcoholic, but they feel there is no choice, that there is no way out. Only escape through the numbing effect of alcohol to cover possible feelings of guilt and the apparent easy solution of denial. Alcoholism and its definition are irrelevant and empty terms.

Alcoholism isn't even defined by the amount a person drinks, but by the effect drinking has on any area of someone's life, such as:

• Arguments with family and friends about how much someone should drink

• Lying or hiding your drinking habits

• Needing a drink so you can relax

• Not remembering what you did during a drinking session (black out)

• Rather spending money on alcohol than on food

• Drinking to feel better about yourself

• Drinking more than you intended to on a regular basis

• Drinking while you know it can be physically dangerous, like drinking and driving

• Neglecting your responsibilities at home and/or at work

• Using alcohol as a self-medication for other health problems, such as anxiety, depression, etc.

• Relying on alcohol to function

• Feel physically compelled to have a drink, for example shaking.

For someone who can recognise him or herself in one or more of the above-stated behaviours the definition of alcoholism is not so relevant. What is important is understanding and the realisation that alcoholism is about pain and frustration, about living a lie, about insecurity and overcoming obstacles, but above all, about human beings.

FACTS ABOUT ALCOHOL

Findings in case of alcoholics differ from person to person. Mostly, the level of consumption of alcohol determines certain features about an alcoholic. Basically alcoholism is a constant disorder, which is accompanied with habitual consumption of alcohol causing serious damage to person's health and mind. Even social and professional activities are deteriorated due to alcoholism habit.

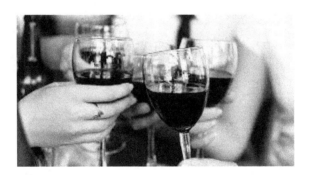

Symptoms

Some familiar symptoms of alcoholism include continuous craving for alcohol, physical dependence on others, loss of memory, loss of appetite and numbness in body parts. This is an accepted fact about alcohol that if once you get into the grip of alcoholism, then in spite of strong urge to keep yourself away from it, it is difficult to do it. You always try to stop drinking but you do not find yourself capable of doing it and at the end you resort back to alcohol. Your alcohol tolerance level needed for extended amount of alcohol increases every time you go for drinking.

Factors Responsible for Alcohol Abuse

There are many factors responsible for alcoholism which includes social causes, environmental reasons and most importantly genetic causes. Generally, the disease of alcoholism is not dependent on the type of alcohol you are consuming, but the factors which affect it greatly include the duration of addiction, quantity of consumption of alcohol and excessive need to consume it. If the alcoholic is in first stage then it is easy to recover from but when it gets into final stage it is very hard to recover without sufficient medical prescription and supervision.

Myth about Alcohol

There are many health related facts about alcoholism. Excess consumption of alcohol leads to grave health problems. If you have recently taken to the alcohol you might suffer from problems like vomiting, loss of appetite, nausea, dizziness and gradually the loss of memory. If you continue it in long terms then you might have to undergo depression, liver cirrhosis, injury to liver, heart failure and failure of central nerve system.

You can easily understand the facts about alcoholism right from the initial warnings and symptoms. One known and popular fact about alcoholism is that it is a kind of drug addiction which can be physical and psychological. Facts about alcoholism are integrated with severe realities that alcoholism is a main cause for decreased activity level and energy amount in the body. It increases the sense of insecurity in alcoholic and affects his or her body system. It can even result in gastrointestinal tract irritation which might be accompanied with corrosion of the esophagus, fatigue, vomiting and stomach linings.

Many other facts about alcoholism are that alcoholism and caffeine are the most widely abused substance, according to a recent research. But on account of alcohol related accidents it is considered more severe problem. There are two ways of alcohol consumption; one is alcohol abuse and the other is alcohol dependence. Alcohol dependence is most harmful as its consequences are characterized by forbearance and withdrawal. Tolerance or forbearance means increased curiosity to drink more for extra intoxication. Withdrawal symptoms appear after discontinuing the regular intake of alcohol. Alcohol abusers are those alcoholics who often drink heavily and then get involved in problems like accidents and missing work.

There are a number of facts associated with alcohol which can drastically affect not only your social life but your work also. If you are aware about these facts then you can save yourself from many grave problems.

ALCOHOLISM RECOVERY

It is easier to develop an addiction to alcohol than it is to recover from alcoholism. Understanding and accepting this, is among the many first steps towards a successful journey towards recovery from alcohol addiction.

There are many obstacles that can actually prevent a person from successfully recovering from alcohol addiction, and you might be surprised to know some of these hurdles.

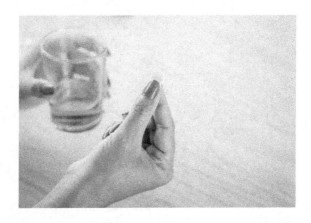

Obstacle 1: Believing that recovery from alcoholism is easy

Through hindsight, it may seem much easier. However while you are going through the fight against alcohol addiction, it will feel like one of the hardest things you have ever had to face. For that matter, it probably is. There is more to recovering from alcohol dependency than just quitting drinking. You may have heard that a recovering alcoholic is always a recovering alcoholic, and that is because recovery is a journey without end.

Overcoming this obstacle:

Before you can fight alcoholism, and win, you have to be prepared to fight. In order to do this, you have to have a full understanding of what you are up against. With the right motivation, it can be easy to make it through each day, taking one step at a time (at your own comfort level) until you are ready to jump in and take back control of your life.

Obstacle 2: Believing that "alcoholism" just means you drink too much

There are many different forms of alcohol dependency. In some cases, a victim drinks every day all day, and in some cases an addict drinks in "binges". You might even be surprised to know that habitual drinking (the habit of drinking at certain times or occasions, including to celebrate or to mourn) is a form of alcohol dependency. Alcohol addiction, no matter what form it is, is not something cut out of stone. The symptoms of alcoholism vary from one individual to the next.

Overcoming this obstacle:

If you have considered quitting drinking, chances are you are suffering alcohol dependency. If alcohol has caused any problems in your life, and you are now conscious of the effects of alcohol in your life; then you are certainly ready to leap over this obstacle and recover from your dependency of alcohol.

Obstacle 3: Believing you can recover from alcoholism on your own

Many have tried and very, very few have been successful. If you really want to recover, you have to really face this fight against alcoholism realistically.

Overcoming this obstacle:

The hardest part is admitting to yourself that you are no longer in control. Whatever form your alcohol dependency has taken, alcohol has taken over. Admitting that you need help is not a sign of weakness; rather it is a great action of personal strength. More importantly, it is the most important action you can take towards recovering from alcohol addiction.

Beginning recovery from alcohol addiction

Your recovery from alcohol addiction begins at an alcohol treatment center. An alcohol rehab is your training base for the battle against alcohol dependency. Here you will find the many tools needed to fight off triggers.

Alcohol Detoxification

Cleansing the body of toxins is the kick start to moving on with your life. It is a lengthy, difficult, and often painful experience that can be nearly impossible to make it through alone. Alcohol detoxification at an alcohol rehab offers professional medical staff, 24/7, with the experience needed to help you through your withdrawal symptoms and back into a healthy body.

Counseling at an Alcohol Rehab Center

As mentioned previously, alcohol dependency takes on many forms. It is also not a matter of "drinking too much". Alcoholism is a disease, and often the symptom of another disease depression. Without qualified counseling at an alcohol treatment center, the underlying disorder is likely to continuously feed to a dependency on alcohol. The result? Continuously repeating the cycle of alcohol dependency.

An alcohol rehab counselor will treat both depression and alcoholism, so when you complete your alcohol rehab program you will be completely stronger and happier, inside out. More importantly, you will be ready for those triggers when they arise.

After an alcohol addiction treatment center

Just as your journey officially begins with alcohol detoxification, it is after you complete your program at an alcohol addiction treatment center that your journey continues. Armed with the tools to recognize triggers and fight urges, you will be back in control. The most important thing to understand that recovering from alcohol dependency is an action, and not just a simple process with a definitive ending.

Is Alcoholism Caused By Genetics or By the Environment?

Genetic and Environmental Factors

According to the National Institute on Alcohol Abuse and Alcoholism (NIAAA), a person's risk of developing alcoholism is 60% determined by his or her genetics and 40% caused by his or her environment. Assuming that these statistics are accurate, what can be done to reduce the chances of becoming addicted to alcohol?

Genetic Causes of Alcoholism

Regarding the genetic determinants of alcoholism, those who say, "nothing can be done" are not totally correct. True, a person cannot change his genetics. Knowing, however, that there is a history of alcoholism in a person's family, for example, can help a person "prevent" this potential problem from ever starting if he practices total abstinence. This kind of preventative thinking is an example of a "proactive" approach to problem solving.

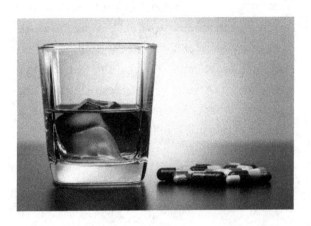

More Proactive Problem Solving

The following illustration, however, is an even more extreme example of "proactive" problem solving that can affect the genetic basis of alcoholism. Maria, a young lady who drinks very infrequently, starts to date a young man named Kirk. As their relationship develops, Maria starts to notice that Kirk gets drunk on a regular basis. In fact, Kirk gets intoxicated at least two or three nights every week. What is especially problematic about Kirk's drinking is that he gets angry and combative when he drinks excessively. On numerous occasions, Maria has tried to encourage Kirk to seek professional help, but each time she starts to discuss his drinking, Kirk gets extremely defensive, starts yelling at her, and then goes to a bar to drink with his buddies. After a year of riding an emotional roller coaster, experiencing numerous hurtful arguments, and going through many difficult alcohol-related situations, Maria finally decides to break up with Kirk. What were the major factors for the breakup? Maria wants to have children and can't see having them with a violent and angry man who is so dependent on drinking alcohol. Moreover, Maria figured that since Kirk is exhibiting such irresponsible behavior in a dating relationship, he could possibly get even worse if they were to get married.

In this illustration, by breaking up with Kirk, Maria has stopped a negative cycle from going any further. Stated differently, by deciding to end her relationship with Kirk, Maria "prevented" the genetics part of the equation from ever becoming an issue.

Concerning Alcoholism, Age Matters

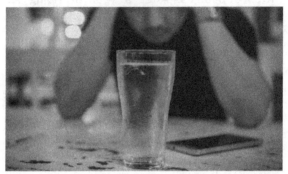

Another important alcohol-related statistic articulated by the NIAAA is that the earlier a person starts drinking alcohol, the more likely she will continue to drink her entire life. This being the case, it therefore makes sense to look for ways that will significantly reduce alcohol abuse by teens, preteens, and by young adults.

An Environmental Framework

Employing an "environmental" approach (as opposed to a genetics-based methodology), higher education seems to be a logical starting point for ways to reduce alcohol problems manifested by our youth. Indeed, since many teenagers go to college and because teen alcohol abuse IS a serious health risk, it is relevant to ask what college administrators can do to significantly reduce student alcohol abuse, especially when teenagers are some of the main "offenders." It is suggested that the following reactive and proactive measures help address this issue.

Reactive and Proactive Measures to Help Reduce Student Alcohol Abuse

• Establish immediate consequences for excessive drinking.

• Discipline repeat alcohol abuse offenders.

• Monitor the drinking activities in the sororities and fraternities.

• Notify parents about their children's drinking activities.

• Talk to the owners of local drinking establishments so that minors and/or intoxicated students are not served alcohol.

• Eliminate mixed messages about alcohol (for instance, removing alcohol advertisements from stadiums and from sports brochures).

• Inform and educate students about the long-term negative consequences of alcohol abuse.

• Increase the number of alcohol-free social and recreational activities that are attractive to students.

Generalizing the Results

With additional effort and some more thought, it seems reasonable to think that alcoholism experts and college administrators will be able to generate even more ways to effectively reduce alcohol abuse at institutions of higher education. Once this is accomplished, moreover, perhaps their findings can be adapted so that they will "work" in other institutions such as junior and senior high schools, boy scouts, girl scouts, churches, camps, and so on.

What is Alcohol Addiction? Alcohol Addiction Counseling and Treating Alcohol Addiction

The alcohol addiction counseling that is available today is much further advanced than the primitive approach used previously for treating alcohol addiction.

Alcohol addiction has existed for many years and is widely known as "alcoholism". Drinking, occasional overindulgence and getting a little 'merry' is nothing new, but most individuals do not take their drinking to the level of alcoholism. Those that do however, frequently see their lives falling apart and, all too often, find themselves in an early grave.

Until the establishment of Alcoholics Anonymous, a non-profit fellowship of recovering alcoholics trying to stay sober one day at a time, there was not much hope for those in the grips of severe alcoholism.

Most alcoholics were bundled off to mental institutions to go through delusion tremors (DTs) - a dangerous state which the body goes into during alcohol withdrawal - or forced into religion as a cure for their problem. Yet none of these 'cures' helped. As soon as the alcoholic would leave the institution or be alone, even for the shortest while, their return to drinking would be quick and imminent.

ALCOHOLISM AS A DISEASE

Thankfully, a lot more is understood about alcoholism in the present day. Although some specialists differ in schools of thought, it is widely believed to be an incurable disease that can be helped by alcohol addiction counseling.

The disease is said to be progressive and fatal, yet can be arrested if the alcoholic ceases to drink and remains abstinent. Because of the disease of alcoholism, an alcoholic cannot stop through their own will, even when their only wish is be abstinent. However, it is possible for someone without the disease to act in a way where their alcohol consumption is too much over a long period, but they are able to stop when they feel that enough is enough. The alcoholic cannot. Many people resort to alcohol to 'drown' their sorrows, but it is only the alcoholic who will carry on for years possibly and will only be able to stop through getting necessary help.

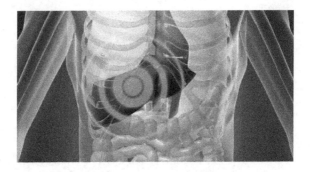

Some believe that people are born alcoholics and that once the first drink is consumed, they begin the slide down the slippery slope descending into alcoholism. Many ask "how does one catch the disease of alcoholism?" No one can be sure, some say that it is hereditary and genetic, some say that it is appropriated through childhood problems, some say that it is a combination of the two.

The Symptoms of Alcoholism

The symptoms of alcoholism vary according to the stage to which the alcoholic has progressed. Some alcoholics may not have progressed to the stage of needing to drink in the morning or to steal to fund their habit. But never the less, if the disease is present, they are a ticking time bomb.

A person who plans to have one drink and eventually drinks ten in one night is not necessarily an alcoholic, although this is a major symptom. The inability to have control over one's drinking once one drink has been consumed is a key symptom of alcoholism.

There is a saying which says "one is too many and a thousand is never enough." This could not be truer for an alcoholic. Usually the alcoholic will have some form of control if they are completely abstinent from alcohol or any other mind or mood altering substances. However, once one drink is consumed, all control is lost and what was intended to be an innocent drink turns into a binge lasting weeks, even months and years.

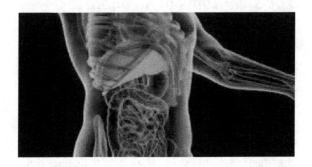

The main symptoms of alcohol addiction are obviously a vast consumption of alcohol, especially at strange times of day and at inappropriate times. An alcoholic who has reached full mental and physical dependence will suffer from DT's when without a drink. Morning tremors are a big sign of a problem and are usually followed by a drink or many to stop the shaking and hysteria, allowing the alcoholic to function on a minimal level. Secretive drinking, lying about consumption and extremely unreliable behaviour are also key warning signs that someone may be an alcoholic. Individuals may be prone to major depression, violence and extremely unstable behaviour accompanied by huge character changes.

THE TREATMENT OPTIONS

Treating alcohol addiction should not only deal with the symptoms, i.e. the drinking. The drinking is not the root problem. It is a symptom. The problem sits within the alcoholic themselves, not in the alcohol.

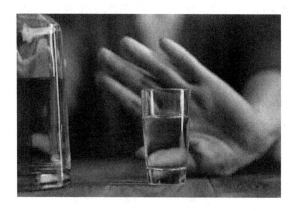

Rehabilitation centres are a good place for an alcoholic to receive treatment, provided they offer individual therapy, group therapy and a programme of recovery so that the alcoholic may remain abstinent when they leave.

Many treatment centres encourage patients to work a twelve step programme, such as the one offered by Alcoholics Anonymous. This programme offers a daily programme of recovery based on working the twelve steps. The twelve steps encourage spirituality, not religion. The twelve step programme's main foundations are staying sober one day at a time, attending meetings, working with a sponsor (a more experienced member of the fellowship), service, literature and trusting in a higher power.

Another key aspect of recovery is a healthy body. Proper diet and regular exercise is very important to a recovering alcoholic's well-being. After years of incredibly unhealthy habits and brutal treatment of their bodies, an alcoholic will feel great improvements in mood and overall well-being.

If an alcoholic can stop drinking, that is the first step towards recovery and abstinence. However, stopping drinking is just the start to arresting this cunning and powerful disease.

Alcoholism can be fatal if not addressed and will get progressively worse. Alcohol addiction counselling, therapy, healthy living and a programme of recovery are the best chance an alcoholic has of recovering. However, at the end of the day, it is the alcoholic's choice to recover and follow these steps to recovery.

Successfully Overcoming Alcoholism Lies in Addressing Both the Alcohol and the "ism"

You can take the alcohol out of alcoholism but what is left is the "ism" part of this disease. The "ism" part of alcoholism is the psychological and personality issues which go hand in hand with the actual over consuming of alcohol.

How do you know if they are an alcoholic?

The question of whether or not someone is suffering from alcoholism is an age old issue. And the truth is, there is not a hard and fast rule. The best answer anyone has been able to come up with is to look at the behavior and the results, or consequences, of that behavior in and on the individual's life circumstances. Without getting into the entire evaluation process, the three key questions are; one, how much and how often do they drink alcohol. Two, what impact is and has drinking had on their life? And three, when you have a drink (or two) what happens? In other words does the person, once they start to drink alcohol, then end up consuming far more alcohol that they intended? This last question is the disease part of alcoholism. Your body has lost the ability to process alcohol and can no longer tolerate any of it, even in small amounts. Arguments can be made in the age old question of whether it is genetically connected, or not.

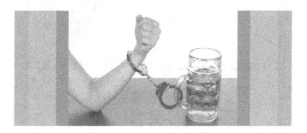

There are a variety of clinical tests, assessments and evaluations which can help determine if a person is drinking behavior has crossed the fine line between heavy drinking and alcoholism. According to Alcoholics Anonymous, only the individual can decide for themselves if they are an alcoholic, or not. Medically speaking, the disease of alcoholism is defined by a type of "allergy" to alcohol. The allergic reaction is triggered by drinking even a small amount of alcohol, which causes the person to then drink a far greater amount of alcohol than they initially intended. The other criteria are the consequences the person has suffered as a result of their drinking behavior.

If drinking has resulted in the loss or damage in some area of their life, it is very likely they are well on their way to being an alcoholic.

The process of recovery from alcoholism

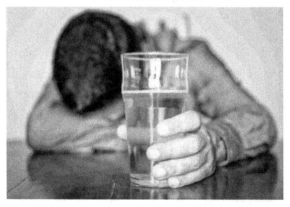

Once someone determines they are alcoholic, the process of addressing it can begin. The first step is getting all the alcohol safely out of their system. This is called detox. Once the person is stable, they should attend alcohol rehab, at some level. Rehab is the educational and therapeutic process of addressing their alcoholism. And begins the process of awakening to their disease and what they need to do to keep it in remission. Going to Alcoholics Anonymous, AA, meetings is considered one of the best ways of both staying abstinent. Some people have been able to simple stop drinking, on their sheer will power, but these cases are rare. Most end up drinking again sooner or later, often with disastrous results.

The "ism" piece

What is this "ism" part of alcoholism? Most alcoholics, for whatever reason, can't seem to cope with the bumpy road of life without drinking considerable amounts of alcohol. This inability to cope with life without alcohol is the "ism" part. Generally, most alcoholics are egotistical and self-centered people. Some are immature, at least for their age. Basically, they use alcohol, which is a drug, to "self-medicate" them as a tried and true method of anesthetizing themselves from the pains of life.

Stopping drinking is never easy, but if an alcoholic is going to stop for good and lead a relatively "normal" life, they need to realize it is process of changing the way they deal with life and all its myriad of problems. It is actually more difficult to heal the "ism" side of the alcoholism problem, but one that must be done successfully if the alcoholic is going to live a good, alcohol-free existence.

ENERGY POINT OF VIEW TO CREATE EMOTIONAL CHOICES

This is an energy point and how alcohol affects a person emotional spirit in their life. There are two parts to this article one is about affects of drinking and how it changes your energy flow through the body and its ability to feel. The second part is how to enhance your emotion spirit force to aid in your recovery.

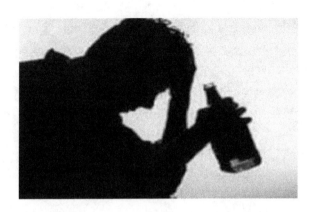

The first part is a review of the affects of drinking alcohol on persons emotional abilities and the affects, on a person's life energy force within their body. The second is how to create choices to overcome the physical, mental and spirit affects of drinking alcohol within your relationships between you and others. Realizing the affects of alcohol in your interactions within yourself and with others and how under the influence, alcohol created judgment that has to be undone and then replaced so a person in recovery can be warmer to others as an expression and receive warmth. To recover from alcohol is about becoming stronger mentally, physically and spiritually that changes a persons emotional connection to them self and their feeling connection to others that is no longer base on past judgment that was developed under alcohol.

Giving up alcohol judgment with its develop emotional connection is painful for the change leaves a hole in a persons history of development of enjoyment for them self. Making a hole in your past from not drinking is a challenge and full of regrets but being in the now and creating your spirit being projected to others that comes back to you in the most positive way through interaction is worth it to others and yourself. Strength in your spirit is the primary force to connect to the body then to the mind so you can feel within your behavior without alcohol. Realizing spirit is the greatest damage from alcohol and its the hardest to understand and realize the effects in recovery. Most people do not work directly to strengthen spirit force but it is done more indirectly within doing other things to recover your God give spirit. Having clarity of the spirit force and how it comes together as force of action when a person is working in the here and now.

To recover is bring the level of ones strength between minds, body and spirit which is breath to higher level bring about a strong sense of the mind and body connection within interaction with others. The affect of ones breath forming ability cannot be over stated to understand the need to develop core/breathing in its many forms to offset the physical cell damage from alcohol and change old habits. Finding ways to increase the bodies ability to feel in its many forms, affects a person ability to change to be positive in their life and express it and be close emotionally to others through judgment.

First thing is an understanding of the physical changes that occur as person drinks and slowly become drunk which in time, if repeated turns into a habit where person feels the need for alcohol. There are so many reasons people develop the taste for alcohol given how many different types of alcohol. Within each person the affects of consuming alcohol affects their body differently, which conditions the mind within the act of drinking to the emotions the body is producing that goes with the events that surrounds person that their emotions attach too. When drinking alcohol during social events or seating home and watching TV or just listening to music affects your energy production by lower it which changes the level of feeling ability to be lower. Drinking alcohol lowers the bodies ability to work with its physical energy and the affects persons physical strength which affects your bodies ability to feel physically.

One of the reasons people drink is to lower physical stress in the shoulders and relaxes the body then mind. Alcohol alters a person sense of being while they are interacting with others around them and this interaction is the foundation to become addicted for ones stress is lower through alcohol but its not real without alcohol so the person does not control of stress but a drug does. Changing ones feeling of stress or sense of emotional weakness that comes with stress feeling that are base on ideas within thoughts that person has learned with drinking alcohol. Responsibilities in life is a big emotional deal and how person view it comes with how they learned it and if alcohol was part of growing up and person learning how to deal with emotions then it a hard road not to drink.

Alcohol influences the physical bodies chemistry down to the level of the cells, where a persons energy productions and the ability of energy flowing through the cells are restricted (the influence of alcohol at the cell level in relationship to energy flowing in a complex one. On one hand it restricts flow but on the other hand it affect energy flow in another way where it enhance flow. Energy flow is pressure and when there is restriction it finds other why to move which create new channels for energy for energy flow, that are not normal. Ones energy force is on going and has to be channeled in some way or reduced). Because of alcohol affecting cells ability to transmit energy which has a long term emotional retarding affect within persons behavior and mental emotional state. Alcohol is a numbing chemical which affects your energy and as you drink and the more you drink the greater the affect on your spirit. Energy and spirit are interlink with breathing and alcohol affects your ability to breathe and that affects your emotional ability for emotional attachment. Alcohol makes person self centered emotionally around his alcohol where others take a back seat to his bottle of alcohol for its what he worships with his spirit of life.

Alcohol emotionally replaces people and becomes a persons emotional attachment and all other people serve that attachment to the alcoholic. To a alcoholic, alcohol is the emotional center to their life and it just come first in thoughts and behavior and emotional attachment. They have only one emotional love and that is alcohol and they are trap in their behavior driven by alcohol. They will spend hours in bar drinking which replaces personal responsibility to family. People in the family have to adjust to the alcoholic emotional demands which is to serve them when they are drunk. You can not trust a drunk for their words are meaningless because their words are in the spirit of alcohol.

When a person becomes alcoholic they replace their God given spirit with the alcohol induce spirit. To recover its about finding ideas and techniques that make your spirit stronger so it can replace the learned alcohol behavior spiritual. What makes alcohol so damaging is within 24 hours its out of the system but the damage on the cell level does not repair it self over time and the emotional damage stays on.

The emotional develop expression at social event under the influence of alcohol can not be repeated with out alcohol so it create a real social emotional conflict on not know how to act and feel at the same time to enjoy the event. So when your having fun and enjoying them self and consuming alcohol, the affects how you relate to your self having fun will be different then if you never taken a drink. For it changes your ability to feel within an event and then leaves a imprint on your being that can not be repeated with out drinking alcohol. So your developing a alcohol spirit in having fun and your God given spirit is not part of the fun and enjoyment. Your creating two different emotional realities, one with out alcohol and one with alcohol. Keep that in mind for recovery, for you have to train your mind, body and spirit to be one person creating your emotional reality when your at a fun event and interaction with others.

Alcohol bonds with water, so alcohol will be part of every cell in the body, to some level. Since alcohol bonds with water so it affects electrical ability of the cells by lessening energy flow through which as the affect of lower your physical feeling ability. The long term affect of consuming alcohol is cell dehydration were its ability to transmit energy flow slows down or not at all and that affect makes a person emotionally cold for they will live in the past. There is no real benefit to long term drinking but a huge lose of life experiences and emotional reality experience abilities. Your life spirit is replaced over time where your world moves around your addiction to alcohol for its your first emotional love for its emotionally comforting.

Here is rule, the younger a person starts to drink the greater the emotional damage and ability to relate to others emotionally and them self within the interaction. You damage your God give spirit by replacing it with the alcohol spirit and that becomes your purpose of life.

Alcohol affects your judgment abilities thereby it affects your purpose in life. If drinking alcohol affects judgment then your decisions are base around alcohol influences that affects emotional judgment and attachments with person emotional spirit. Making enough judgments under the influence of alcohol it become your process to judging thinking around you and emotional relationships. If something affects your judgment and you act on that judgment it becomes your emotional reality. When you physically act on your judgment your acting in emotional way so your decision become your emotions and that will be you. So what you express when you are drunk that is you now but repeated enough that will be you all the time even when your not drunk. The term dry drunk comes into play here, that is the long term affect of drinking.

The physical, mental and spiritual damage that is caused by drinking alcohol can be seen around you in movies and if you look to books there are so many of them on alcohol and the damage. There is information on alcohol and its damage to families, physical health is so large it is not reasonable to drink. But drinking is an emotional venture, it changes your normal emotional spirit and that is the power of the experience of drinking alcohol.

The second part is how to make your physical energy spirit stronger within your program to recover your God give spirit and purpose. How much physical damage has been done to the body and brain affects the physical part of recovery but the spirit recovery has no limits. Do not under estimate your power to change your judgment and your emotional abilities and enjoyment what you have now by developing your spirit for that can help over come regret. Life is about what you creating now and how you are enjoying and developing the emotional content within your responsibilities that you chose to create. The old saying, it is not about what you have but what you over came in life that is valuable. Life is a challenge to work and develop your emotional spirit within what you do in life with your responsibilities to live.

When a person choose to change from the alcohol emotional spirit behavior, they are going on a emotional journey that is challenging and there has to be a program to give values or relearn values to create from your emotional energy spirit. To replace their alcoholic emotional spirit by recovering your own God given spirit, begins with understanding at some level the emotional physical spirit damage. Finding ideas, concepts and techniques, methods that affect their personal emotional spirit reality and then develop it, into their life that replaces the alcohol emotional spirit. Change is about replacement and not just reacting to it. Programs are key component for person to learn to change and making good choices and develop emotional values. Finding the programs that affect you takes judgment to use the ideas within each program to change your values to life and emotional behavior to your self and others for keep in mind its about interaction and the emotional feeling being projected during the interaction.

This program is to add to all of the other programs that work on aiding person to make judgment decisions with out alcohol influence and feel the physical spirit that is you and what you work from in life. Realizing your a physical spirit being by feeling the flow of energy through out your body is experience that can be repeated but will always feel and be different for person is more then they think in thoughts. First realization is the force within the power of core/breathing that goes to and relate to person internal force development that engages the mind and body coordinating connection. Look to breathing forms as force that works from the internal side of person with the mind and body for to create the breath is working the torso to some level and the more you work the torso the more energy force.

This program is about creating emotional choices by using your spirit to affect the brain and body to change your emotional reality connection to life interaction with others and yourself. Drinking is choice in the beginning but then turns into a compulsion. Your emotional spirit has changed for what is a compulsion, but a lot of energy build up in the body and then it is releases through behavior with alcohol and then relaxation and calmness. Keep in mind the word calmness for recovery for with calmness new direction will be seen and realized and developing techniques that create emotional, physical state of calmness gives clarity in ones emotional state. Meditation and through some form of meditating for short period of time each day and in some way creates calmness that affect persons judgment abilities and can be refined so new judgment direction can be seen. Part of recovery is develop ways to create calmness where thoughts are second to feeling physically and projecting calmness. Calmness has to be projected to be affective in changing a persons emotional states. Just developing calmness for short period of time is nice and helpful but only when person realizes ability to project calmness is the full affect of that state of being, can be felt and used in life. The old saying when you use something then you know it then. Otherwise calmness is thought process and is not part of persons emotional make up everyday.

Keep in mind, alcohol is defined as spirits in licenses to sale alcohol for when you drink you replace your spirit with the alcohol spirit. Here is question for people that are starting to drink. What would you lose as an experience of life, if you never taken a drink of alcohol in your life. Then what will you gain if you drink is the other side of the question? To be real about your decision to drink or not to drink, look at the affects of people that have become addicted to alcohol so if you drink, your taking a risk that you can become addicted to alcohol. So drinking alcohol is a physical, mental and emotional risk to become addicted to alcohol with all the loses to your self and others around you. To be a alcoholic just does not affect one person but it hurts other people that care and love you. All alcohol does is lowers the ability to feel and think within events of life and your spirit to life. You just do not do has much in life emotionally with alcohol as your spirit. Remember your a spirit being within a physical body creating choice to develop one self and realize your life.

If you have fallen to alcohol and have become alcoholic and have made the choice to change the challenge is creating choices to develop your emotional behavior reality judgment in your everyday interaction with others. Finding ideas, concepts and methods that have physical techniques that helps you recover from the physical and emotional damages of consuming alcohol and your loss of your ability to love. Only with your own spirit can you love and find the emotional behavior that projects your feeling around you and that takes time and effort to learn how to feel again. Alcohol has damage their body to feel warmth from others so the mind makes up things.

Approach to recovery from alcohol, and even other drugs, has to be a blend of three primal forces that interact that gives us are abilities to be emotional spirit creative beings. The three basic element words are mind, body and spirit within a persons behavior. Alcohol affects all three elements that composes the creative personality and their ability to create their emotional reality in life. There is no emotional life out side of alcohol for the alcoholic that is reality.

The most powerful ideas and concepts to affect recovery and enhance persons emotional attachment to life is around the development of a persons spiritual forces within, to be express through emotional behavior. Through spiritual development affects and influence emotional ideas in the mind (that has been damage from alcohol judgment) that affects decision in physical development and emotional behavior. One of the great forces of being a spiritual being is are ability to pray and feel the affects within a prayer. How you pray within prayer is a force that affects person sense of life and recovering a person spirit of being emotional with judgment and development to others. Praying is natural for its a spirit ability and finding the way to pray is learned to affect energy flow and feeling within prayer which setup the level positive force to feel physically.

Realize the physical damage caused by drinking and being drunk and becoming a alcoholic takes lot of work to recover your energy abilities again to a level that lets a person create emotional attachments out side the range that alcohol limits them. This is physical work, directed by the mind that affects energy production and flow that lets the body feel again with person spirit. Enhancing your physically feeling ability is part of recovery and it takes lot of mental focus to reconnect the mind to the body, then expressing that feeling which is creating new emotional energy channels in physical exercise and walking. Walking is natural act that reflects a person emotional state for people walk with emotions being projected through feelings of the body movement. How you walk is big deal and changing how you walk is changing your emotional feeling being projected. There is sad, mad and happy walking movement that others can see for your projecting these emotional states through movement of the body during walking. So walking and creating a new emotional state to be projected is experience of development.

Suggestion; understand the word spirit from a mental point of view, a physical point of view and energy point of view for it takes all of them to bring human spirit into focus and use. Each point of view has to be seen connected to the other in order to be useful in recovery from alcohol. If you take recovery from alcohol as a personal adventure into truth and responsibility that develops their personal emotions spirit through testing them self in the most positive way, so person realize and develops judgment with action to others and them self.

Note about aging, the older you get the future become less and your mentally relive your past. So what you have done and what you over came in life, either will put smile on your face or sadness will be your everyday feeling. The more and hard you work to create your emotional development can be, if directed effectively will create rewards far above what you think now. Finding methods that affect you in your stages of recovery and personal development take judgment base on purpose. Here is the question and the clearer you have of the answer the more affective within time spent. What emotional reality do you want to create within your self and while interaction with other on daily bases with the time you have left in life.

The word spirit is rooted in the word breath, breathing and to breathe for its energy that composes a persons spirit. The ideas of a persons spirit has history connection to breath and breathing and understanding this history creates choices to affect ones spirit physically. There is Qi Gong, Chic Gong and Zen breathing all relates to the development of spirit by shaping persons breathing and person directive mental state. Singing affects persons spirit to recover from alcoholism. There is whole lot of ideas to explore that can affect you in energy and spirit that lets person to become stronger. Ideas of being are very much parts of recovery for they have to fill your head with life and about life and people that love you. You learn about your self through others around you otherwise you do not know yourself.

Here is rule if you want to recover from alcoholism. You change through becoming stronger physically internally through breath development and energy flow that affects your emotional abilities. Being clear here, it is physical strength internally from the core and breathing from the core movement, a person needs to change to affect emotions within the development of strength from within your internal feeling that sets up the affects of changing to be positive that over comes the affects from being a alcoholic which is negative in feeling development and connection. Internal strength exercises to become emotionally stronger enhances a person ability to be positive and enjoy their life and being a human being. judgment and better judgment to become morally stronger comes with being physically stronger within what you due daily in life interacting with others. Here is internal fact, negative emotions will make the body weak. One reason is it change persons breath range and makes it shorter and with less breath less endurance.

The power of core/breathing is central for strength that let person have more choices to create and develop their emotional connection to physical movement. As a exercise walking can be an experience that let a person enhance their physical connection to the mental emotional state by changing stress in shoulder and tension in muscles feeling through out the body while walking. Change your stress and you change your emotional reality. So you have to find techniques that affect stress in shoulders that free up energy and affect the flow energy in the body to enhance feeling.

The approach for males to recover from alcoholism is different then from females for the end is the same but the approach to be affective should be look at differently. Example is males are physical to emotional and females are emotional to physical, so strength is the key but its two different type of development with emotional attitudes within the development of physical exercise to connect to emotional feeling within the body

I like to introduce and new idea or concept to aid person to recover from alcohol addiction within their program. This is base on energy point of view. People have three energy flowing channels and how you affect one influence the other two. There is what you can see the nerves system. The next is what you can not see the acupuncture system or the pressure points through out the body that affect energy flow and feeling and health. The new idea that person can play with to aid in recovery is created by the person them self. I call it the physical emotional energy channels that person use to express their emotional state all the time. Person learns to develop their emotional physical energy channels to express their emotions to other around them and other read them. When you change your emotional energy channels you change your feeling about interaction with life. Walking is emotional event so how you walk is reflection of your emotion mood in the now. Person as the ability to create their emotions and then express it by feeling their body in walking. It is not the only way to affect person emotional energy channels.

Emotional energy channels is physical and its on going with your body tension emitting energy directed by your mental state. Ones emotional energy channel shapes a persons physical body and its movement is to project emotional energy around them. How you shape your body affects your emotional projection ability so by changing your body shape that affects muscle tension within that shape and through core/breathing and mind creating attitude, a person can create a different emotional reality experience within that new shape. This idea uses mind, body and breath, energy build to spirit as a strengthening force to give person a choices to change once they know what to change too.

The development of powerful breathing from the core which affects the whole torso and expands range within the torso that affects persons emotional strength. It is torso strength that is the primary strength then arms and hands and legs and feet. But it all begins in the center of your body and the center of the core. Energy and strength are connected and begins in the center of the core and then goes up to the arms and head or down to legs, feet and toes. The mind directs the energy and strength that the core produces.

The more you move the core to create your breath the greater your physical strength and energy for you are lessening atrophy of the muscles within the torso. Look at your breathing in different emotional states. Breathing is a support of your emotional state so how you change your breathing during events in life affects your emotional reality.

There is so much more about a person spirit, so keep a open mind with judgment and purpose and do not waste your time and energy in life its short in supply. Warning: Be careful what you ask for, you may get it.

This program and ideas is base on the fact that humans are a spiritual being having a human experience. By being spiritual being, people can create choices within their spirit through their interaction in life and their purpose and judgments. Keep in mind spirit is only one part interacting with the other two parts. Mind, body and spirit (breath and energy). The importance of developing core/breathing to enhance person internal connection to mind and body and strength physically and emotionally should be a major part of recovery for its the spirit side of change in life.

After many years of teaching at a drug rehab, my program of stress management to replace addiction impulse and seeing people leave the program in good mental and physical shape but then seeing them back after a few month, in the program gave rise to some questions. The question is what is the problem that a person has to realize so they can create a different emotional reality force that is more powerful then their drug emotional development. It is balance of mind, body and spirit and realizing humans are spiritual being looking for ways to develop their spirit force of life. The word LOVE is only one example of the emotional reality that only humans can create as bond between others that reflects the human spirit. Drugs damages the bodies ability within energy flow and feeling that affect a person spirit force in life for it affects breathing ability. Finding techniques to affect ones spirit that over comes the damage that drugs has caused, that affects persons abilities in life to feel and project a large range of feeling take lot of work within the mind, body and spirit connecting together. In todays culture drugs are a powerful personal force and causes much damage to a person spirit in life but its just a challenge to create emotional reality and overcome and realize their own personality within their short period of time in life. Just using mental reasoning base on drugs are bad, and you have emotional conflicts all mental base ideas, that are need, but they do not directly affect persons spirit only the mind and some what the body. Drug attack the spirit of person the most and affect the body and mind for under the influences of drugs person form judgment that affect their life. Releasing old drug emotional reality is PAINFUL experience and also needs replacement to it. Drug addiction is a spiritual set back and unless that is address all reasoning will fail to change person behavior and emotional reality only when reasoning is connected to spirit does it have driving force of action and reality. The first part of recovery should be centered around spirit and being a spiritual being and how drug reality changes it and the great lose happens within person.

IMPACT OF ALCOHOL ON DOMESTIC VIOLENCE

Intoxication and violence can be a common pairing when you or a loved one starts drinking alcohol. There is never a good excuse to be violent to a loved one, friend and children or pet during an episode of drinking too much alcohol. Unfortunately, these types of occurrences happen quite frequently in the United States, and police are often called to assist in handling the situation. Domestic violence is not acceptable, and can lead to legal and/or medical issues for both you, and the individual you may have harmed.

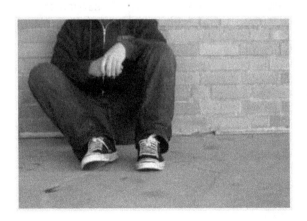

Over time, one of the most common excuses for domestic violence has become, "But I was drunk?" As an unacceptable answer for wrongful action, this type of behavior does come with a plethora of consequences. Additionally, even if one person was throwing punches or yelling, it is also most common that the other individual fighting back, was also intoxicated.

Domestic violence cases also can effect more than just the two or more individuals within the central altercation. When these occurrences do take place, police officers are often called, along with medical assistance for any individual who may have been harmed. Homes can be destroyed, children can be traumatized and in the morning, you may be embarrassed by all that your neighbors have witnessed.

When is it time to make a big change? It is often the case that a cycle becomes relevant with those that drink alcohol and take part in violent activities. After a violent episode, perhaps the couple will make up the next day with apologies? Or, they will each go about their day as if the prior day never happened; walking down the same path again that very same night, thereafter. To get yourself, and your loved one out of this cycle, there is a need to make a big change.

How do I get myself help? If you are suffering from a harmful alcohol addiction, it is best to consult with professionals at a drug and alcohol rehabilitation center. These individuals know exactly what you going through and are able to give expert advice on steps to move you toward a healthy rehabilitation program.

If your spouse, roommate, friend, or otherwise is suffering from an unhealthy addiction to alcohol, you must first remove yourself from the situation. Do not continue to allow yourself to be subjected to bodily and/or verbal abuses. Move in with a family member, or a good friend, temporarily.

Then, see if you can assist your loved one in finding the help that they so desperately need.

Call a rehab center in or out of your area, and collect information today. It's never too late to change the path of addiction, and stop domestic abuse from regularly occurring in your life.

ALCOHOL AND HEALTH EFFECTS OF ALCOHOL ON THE BODY

Alcohol and health effects of alcohol on the body can be short term or long term effects. The consumption of alcohol and health related problems can occur over a short time frame, while other conditions and long term effects of alcohol on the body may only happen following years of alcohol abuse.

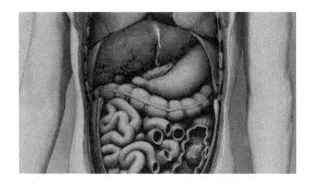

Alcohol comes into direct contact with the mouth, throat, esophagus, stomach and intestines as well as being absorbed into the bloodstream. Health problems can begin as headaches, feeling nauseated, sore throat or indigestion. However, if alcohol abuse continues, these and other alcohol and health symptoms can develop into more serious illnesses and diseases.

Here are examples of short term health effects of alcohol on the body:

• Nausea, Vomiting, Dizziness, Hangovers - excessive alcohol consumption can result in the body trying to protect itself by getting rid of the alcohol and vomiting. Alcohol and health and the central nervous system are related since alcohol affects a person's sense of balance and orientation, leading to a feeling of nausea and/or dizziness. Hangovers are partly due to the body's dehydration caused by alcohol consumption, and hangover effects of alcohol on the body may be felt a few hours after consuming alcohol.

• Loss of Muscle Control - slurred speech is one of the effects of alcohol on the body. Impaired judgment and poor coordination are alcohol and health effects that can lead to falls and accidents.

• Adverse Interactions with Medications - alcohol is known to interact negatively with at least 100 medications. For example, antihistamines taken with alcohol can increase the drowsiness that this medication by itself can cause. Large doses of the painkiller acetaminophen taken together when consuming alcohol increases the risk of liver damage.

• Pregnancy Risks - alcohol can cause numerous birth defects, the most serious being fetal alcohol syndrome. Babies born with fetal alcohol syndrome will have physical abnormalities, mental impairment and problems with behavior. To avoid negative alcohol and health effects during pregnancy, do not drink alcohol while pregnant as no one knows exactly how much alcohol causes birth defects.

Because alcohol and health effects can involve many organs in the body, long-term heavy drinking puts you at risk for developing serious health conditions and illnesses. Here are examples of long term effects of alcohol on the body:

• Liver Inflammation and Cirrhosis of the Liver - liver inflammation symptoms include abnormal yellowing of the skin, eyeballs and urine, fever and abdominal pain. And in the case of cirrhosis, as many as one in five heavy drinkers will develop cirrhosis of the liver. Alcohol is especially harmful to the liver since the liver is needed to metabolize alcohol. Alcohol destroys liver cells, and it destroys the ability of the liver to regenerate new cells.

• Cancer - long term heavy drinkers increase their risk for certain forms of cancer such as cancer of the mouth, throat and esophagus and colon.

• Heart disease - long term heavy drinking increases a person's risk for developing high blood pressure and heart disease.

• Pancreaitis - long term heavy drinking can result in the development of inflammation of the pancreas called pancreaitis. The pancreas is needed for food digestion, and pancreaitis symptoms include severe abdominal pain and weight loss. Pancreaitis can be life-threatening.

Additional long term negative alcohol and health effects on the body include damage to the brain, nerve damage, bleeding in the esophagus, erectile dysfunction in men, insomnia and depression. If you'd like to learn more about alcoholism stages and warning signs, there are proven resources available that can help. It is never too late to begin recovery from alcohol addiction.

How Alcoholism and Hypoglycemia Controls Body, Mind, and Spirit

Alcoholism is a health affliction of the mind, body and soul. Virtually anyone can become an alcoholic if they are around the conditions that breed addictive behavior such as alcoholism - that would be environmentally, physically, emotionally, and spiritually. Alcoholism is an addiction that attaches itself to the body, mind, and spirit of its victims. Let's take a look.

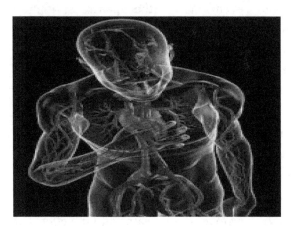

Physical Addiction To Alcohol

The physical addiction to alcohol is an operation that deals with how the pancreas processes sugar in the bloodstream. In the alcoholic/hypoglycemic individual the pancreas does not do a very efficient job in processing the sugars from the alcohol.

Here is how it works: The alcoholic literally craves his first few drinks of alcohol just for the sugar aspect of it. (If there is no alcohol around, he will most likely gorge out on sugar foods to curb his addiction). Once the alcoholic has had his first few drinks it depresses blood sugar levels even more (the pancreas is too overloaded to do its job efficiently)! So the alcoholic craves even more sugar to correct this low blood sugar state and the vicious cycle continues. Brain cells demand more alcohol to replace the lack of sugar. Hence, the alcoholic craves alcohol.

I am a recovered alcoholic of fifteen years and I have done extensive research into the effects of alcoholism on the body and can safely tell you that once diet is improved and hypoglycemia treated through proper diet, the physical addiction for alcohol will subside. When I was an alcoholic/hypoglycemic I would eat sweets and drink Pepsi all day if I didn't have access to alcohol. I was an emotional basket case.

Poor diet is the culprit for physical addiction to alcohol. How do I know this? Because I have listened to my body and I corrected hypoglycemia and physical cravings for alcohol through diet. The best diet for the alcoholic, diabetic, hypoglycemic is a whole grain diet. Throw out all refined food products from your kitchen cupboards and go natural! Foods such as whole wheat bread, brown rice, whole grain pasta, beans, legumes, and oatmeal all work to stabilize and metabolize blood sugar levels, which gives the overloaded pancreas a break so it can start to do its job properly.

Whole grains are best because they are digested slowly into the body system resulting in an optimal environment for blood sugar levels - there is no spiking, no cravings, and no emotional and physical imbalances. Diet plays a huge role in how our brain works. With a whole grain, whole foods diet, the brain stops sending out signals for more alcohol or sugar.

To sum this up I am going to say that alcoholism could very well be a symptom of hypoglycemia. Not all people who have low blood sugar become alcoholics mainly because the rest of the triggers for alcoholism aren't present in that individual.

Psychological Addiction To Alcohol

Now we come to the emotional and mental aspects of alcoholism. Alcoholics usually have emotional ups and downs, are easily agitated, suffer from anxiety and panic, have a low self esteem, and often feel depressed. These symptoms are because they have hypoglycemia. Hypoglycemia is as much an emotional affliction as it is physical. All of the above are symptoms of hypoglycemia or sugar overload syndrome.

Ninety-five percent of alcoholics have low blood sugar. But what happens when there is a change in diet? Is hypoglycemia cured? Yes! But understand, if I deliberately bang my head against the wall several times I'm going to have some bumps and bruises. In the same way if I deliberately eat a poor diet of refined food products my body and mind is going to let me know about it through a vitamin/mineral deficiency. We are in control of what we eat. Your doctor doesn't care what you eat. If you don't do anything about a poor diet your body will.

Most alcoholics have a difficult time managing their emotions or understanding reality. I truly thought I could not cope with life unless I was drinking. I was scared to death to stop drinking! And in a way this is very true for the alcoholic/hypoglycemic because they are so vitamin deficient that their brain works in puzzling ways. It can be a confusing, fearful, and anxious time for the alcoholic when they first get sober...until they begin to take care of their diet! Unless the alcoholic changes their eating habits they will never stay sober because the physical addiction to alcohol is the craving aspect of addiction. If you have ever been addicted to cigarettes than you know what I'm talking about.

Alcohol is the alcoholic's best friend and losing their best friend may mean they will never be able to cope with life on life's terms. Of course, the truth is all alcoholics who become truly sober (not dry drunk) emotionally, physically, mentally and spiritually will look back on their alcoholic days and laugh because they truly can live without alcohol and NEVER CRAVE ALCOHOL OR SUGAR EVER AGAIN! Once diet is corrected and the alcoholic is sober for at least six months he'll begin to realize that he can function just fine without alcohol.

QUIT DRINKING ALCOHOL AND GET BACK YOUR LIFE

Alcoholism is a common problem that many men and women face in the world today. Most of these men and women do not even realize that they have a drinking problem and do nothing about it. If you have decided that you want to quit drinking alcohol, then you have made a wise decision that could save your relationships, your health, and your life. Even if you are not really an alcoholic, you should quit consuming alcohol because alcohol will only harm your health and you might become addicted to it. If you want to learn how to quit drinking alcohol, then you've come to the right place.

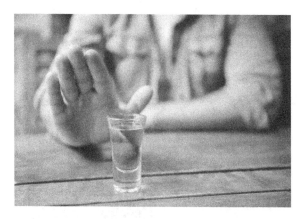

What You Can Do to Quit Drinking Alcohol

In order to quit consuming alcohol successfully, you must first realize and admit to yourself that you are becoming addicted to alcohol and you can't stop drinking it. If you don't admit to yourself that suffering from a disease called alcoholism, then not even the best doctors will be able to treat you. In order to fight it, you must first realize that you have alcoholism. Once you have decided to fight it and quit consuming alcohol, enter an in-patient detoxification program at your local hospital or treatment center.

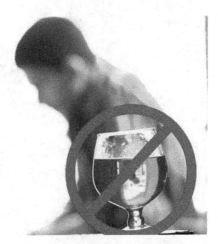

It can take a few days or a whole week for you to complete the entire detoxification process, depending on how addicted you are to alcohol. During this period, you are not allowed to drink alcohol and you will experience some alcohol withdrawal symptoms. If you are severely addicted to drinking, some of the alcohol withdrawal symptoms you might experience are hallucinations and shaking. The medical professionals at the hospital or treatment center can provide medications that reduce the withdrawal symptoms you are experiencing. Entering a detoxification program is the best way to quit consuming alcohol successfully.

TIPS TO QUIT DRINKING ALCOHOL SUCCESSFULLY

If you have severe alcoholism, experts recommend that you undergo therapy in order to deal with any underlying issues that are triggering the urge to drink. A therapist can also teach you how to handle the temptation of taking alcohol. It may also be beneficial if your family included in the therapy because alcohol abuse can affect your entire family. It is recommended that you undergo therapy as soon as you finish your detoxification program so that you don't return to your old drinking habit.

There are some medications can also help you quit consuming alcohol more effectively if you don't want to enter an in-patient detoxification program or undergo therapy. Visit your doctor and ask him about intravenous and oral medications that can help you quit consuming alcohol and avoid relapses. Your doctor may recommend medications that discourage alcohol consumption by making you sick when you drink alcohol. There are also medications that help you quit drinking by reducing the alcohol cravings in your brain. Remember to ask your doctor about these medications before you decide to use them in order to prevent harmful side effects and other health problems.

ALCOHOL AND ANXIETY ATTACKS GO HAND IN HAND

Alcohol and anxiety are inextricably linked for many people. It might come as a surprise, but alcohol is one of the biggest causes of anxiety attacks and panic disorder there is. While many of us use alcohol, in the form of a beer or two, or a glass of wine, to relax after a long and stressful day, doing this can have the opposite effect for a great many people. People drink alcohol and anxiety attacks often follow.

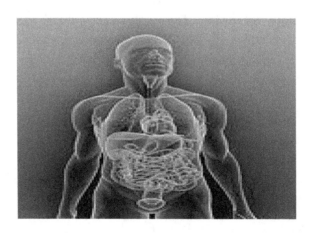

There are thousands of people from all walks of life who like an occasional drink, and indeed, drinking in moderation can provide many benefits. However, the problems start when we begin to overindulge in alcoholic drinks. The body can be affected in many different ways by alcohol abuse; it's not only alcohol and anxiety attacks that are linked. Alcohol can affect your health adversely in many ways, for example it can damage the kidneys and the liver, or it can lead to dependency. It can even affect the way your mind functions.

Drink too much alcohol and you will also find that you are unable to operate to the best of your capabilities. This happens because if you overindulge in alcohol, the feeling that we know as a hangover is actually caused by the nutrients and minerals in your body being diverted to your liver, away from where they should be, because the liver requires them to try and break down the alcohol in your blood stream faster. Along with this feeling of grogginess, drinkers also feel dehydrated from alcohol and anxiety attacks can result from this.

Alcohol and anxiety attack symptoms are basically the same as that of any regular panic attack, with sufferers experiencing the shakes, terrible fear, seating, clamminess and horrible nausea. You may notice that you only have these kinds of attacks after a heavy bout of drinking, or you may at least notice they are more common after such episodes. If so, then alcohol and anxiety are definitely partners here, and so you should cut back on the amount of alcohol you consume to stop panic attacks from happening.

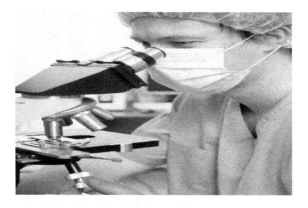

There are a number of medical professionals right now who feel that alcohol and anxiety attack sufferers are usually people who started off with regular panic disorder, and then turned to alcohol as a way of trying to fight these off or otherwise lift their depressive mood. However, drinking alcohol as an anxiety cure is the biggest mistake you can make. People with panic disorders tend to be very susceptible to chemical imbalances in their body, and drinking large quantities of alcohol will cause significant amounts of these, thus exacerbating their panic problems.

Doctors have known about this link between alcohol and anxiety for years now. Over-consumption of alcohol is able to change the chemistry of the brain, enhancing the likelihood of anxious people suffering from panic attacks. And not only is it the drinking that is bad, as alcohol withdrawal can also lead to the same symptoms.

If you suffer from panic disorder and like to have a drink to make you feel relaxed, perhaps you would be better off cutting out the alcohol altogether and seeing if this can help lessen the bad experiences you are having.

ALCOHOL'S EFFECTS IN THE BRAIN

Alcohol can make you laugh or it can make you cry, it can make you lively or make you sleepy, it can boost your confidence or make you act the fool. How can alcohol have all these different effects on people? If we want to know how alcohol affects our moods and behaviors we must first understand a bit about how the brain works.

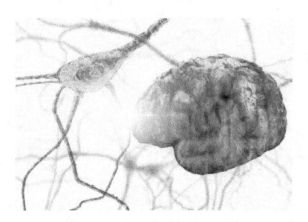

The human brain is made up of about 100 billion nerve cells (also known as neurons). Everything that we think, feel or do is the result of electrical signals passing back and forth between neurons. These electrical signals require the help of chemicals called neurotransmitters in order to pass from neuron to neuron. Scientists have identified around 60 different neurotransmitters so far and tell us that there are probably many more yet to be identified.

Different neurotransmitters have different effects in the brain. For example, serotonin is connected with mood. People suffering from clinical depression tend to have a shortage of serotonin in their brains, and medications like Prozac can help to alleviate depression by increasing the availability of serotonin in the brain. Endorphins are a class of neurotransmitters which act as the brain's natural painkillers.

Electrical signals in the brain are transmitted in the following manner: The neuron which is sending the electrical signal releases a neurotransmitter, and the neuron which is receiving the electrical signal accepts the neurotransmitter at a site which is called a receptor. When the neurotransmitter from the first neuron chemically binds to the receptor of the second neuron the electrical signal is transmitted. Neurotransmitters and receptors work like locks and keys: there is at least one different receptor for each different neurotransmitter. For example, an endorphin receptor can only be triggered by and endorphin, a serotonin receptor can only be triggered by serotonin, and so on. Different neurons have different receptors. Some neurons will only be triggered by serotonin, some only by an endorphin, and so on for all the different neurotransmitters.

The Effects Of Alcohol Abuse Can Be Dramatic And If Left Unchecked Life Shattering

The pressures of life presents us all with trials and tribulations that we need to overcome.. Unfortunately too many of us are now turning to what is perceived to be an instant relief that is found in consuming copious quantities of alcohol. The problem is that the relief is temporary when you wake up the next day you still have the same problems to face. Many people drink, and become alcoholics, to help them to forget their daily problems or even to seemingly ease the emotional pain they may be experiencing in their lives. They seek further solace in the blur of alcoholic haze.

As with the abuse and over indulgence in anything there are effects that appear unexpectedly The effects of alcohol abuse come in many forms. Some are emotional, some are physical, and some can even be financial. The reality is that the negative effects of alcohol abuse far outweigh any supposed benefits you may think that it brings to you.

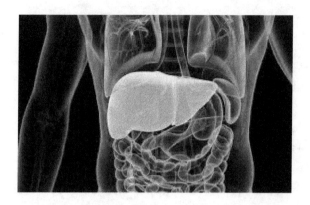

Although the alcoholic may not realize it one of the effects of alcohol abuse is the destruction of your emotional well being. Sometimes alcohol abuse can bring out the worst in a person. This abuse is often directed towards your family and friends who can in most cases be counted on to stand by you in your hour of need. But there is only so much physical and emotional abuse that your family and friends can take before they are forced to turn their back on you.

Usually your friends and family are your support structure; they will stand by you in good times and bad. Alcohol can lead to physically fighting with your friends and family and it can also lead to a loss of trust between you.

Ask yourself how can anyone trust someone that is drunk all the time? Sometimes the results are that your friends and family are either forced to abandon you to avoid you taking them down into your personal hell or they are forced to seek an intervention. Either result puts a great deal of strain on the relationships and can cause serious emotional damage.

Losing It All

When somebody becomes alcohol dependent they often find ways to sneak a drink during their day at work this tends to reduce their productivity and in some cases endanger their being as they try to perform their tasks in an alcoholic stupor. Most, if not all employers will automatically terminate drunk employees. Therefore loss of income is another effect of alcohol abuse and when you lose jobs to the effects of alcohol abuse it unleashes an entire series of terrible events to unfold. At some point you can no longer pay your bills, your home and car get taken away, the family you have sworn to support has to leave to find a better way in life, and you are left with nothing.

It is not an exaggeration to say that if you continue to abuse alcohol on a daily basis that you stand to lose literally everything that you hold dear in your life and your road to recovery will be long and difficult.

Alcohol abuse is everywhere, just look around you and you will see the suffering that it causes. The road to recovery is strewn with alcoholics who's lives have been ruined not to mention all the pain and anguish suffered by family and friends.

Recovery from the effects of alcohol abuse is not as easy as the movies and television make it look. It is a long and painful process. Many people try and fail at many times over before they finally do succeed..

Thankfully there is a way out of this terrible scourge but real strength and determination is required to dig your way out of this quagmire.

ALCOHOL AND TREATMENT CENTER FOR BETTER SURVIVAL

The utilization of addictive substances such as drugs and alcohol has surprisingly increased in the past few years. We are not talking about any particular country. It has become a common scenario of most of the countries of the world. Many researches have already been conduct to witness and compare the addiction statistics of the world. With the increasing number of patients of drugs and alcohol addiction every year, lot of alcohol and drug rehab treatment centers have come into existence to help people suffering from any kind addiction and their families who cannot bear the pain of their dear ones. Their prime concern is to offer a required helping hand to the individuals who are struggling to come over with this dreadful disease.

No doubt in the fact that these alcohol and drug rehab centers are well established with all drug and alcohol addiction treatment services and plays a vital role in turning a life of addicted person back to normal. These rehab centers bring a ray of hope in the lives of addicted people and help them in making their life balanced and productive like before. Yes, it is true that coming over with the trap of drug or alcohol addiction is quite tough. But not losing a hope is what that can actually help an individual in getting out of the trap of alcohol or drug addiction. Thanks to the alcohol and drug rehab treatment centers that are running since long just to make the life of addict's easy living and normal like of other individuals. They offer various drug treatment programs, alcohol treatment programs and dual diagnosis programs that are customized as per the physical and mental condition of the addicted people.

All the treatment programs offered by them are designed to help all those addicted people who want to fight against addiction and live their life in far better manner. Enrolling in alcohol and drug rehab treatment centers is must for the better survival and living of the individuals suffering from the addiction of such heath hazardous substances that are dangerous for life. These days, newly established rehab centers are well equipped with the advance technology and machines so that the best treatment can be offered to the patients. They try to come up with the highly effective programs to control this life infecting disease.

Drug and alcohol addiction is a major issue that have already ruined life of many people and continuing with the same. Such kinds of addiction not only affect an individual but also his or her family as well. It leaves addicts in a shocking stage wherein they cannot decide what is good and what is bad for them. In order to come over with such shock and have a better survival, it is essential to take the addicted person to any best alcohol and drug rehab treatment center surrounded with all the treatment programs and facilities. By taking this wise step, you can give a new life to the people suffering from drug or alcohol or dual addition.

How to Fight Alcoholism?

Alcoholism is not something new to write on. Nevertheless, unfortunately nobody could persuade people to stop drinking. People, who cannot get alcohol due to financial reason or any other reason, sometimes take medicines having alcohol in them. This practice is even more injurious to health.

Alcoholism is very common all over the world. It is very easy to get into it but people find it really hard to get rid of it. Teenagers often start taking alcohol out of fun and excitement. Gradually, they become an addict and when they come to know about this cruel fact, it is already too late. First, they panic, and then they start overlooking the fact from themselves. Later they find it difficult to keep up with their families and thus the battle begins.

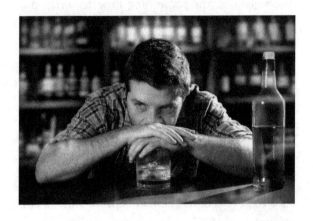

People who get into alcoholism make promises to quit it but they break them as soon as they make them. In this manner they start hurting their self respect along with mental and physical health and start losing their self confidence.

After all this discussion, one starts thinking that is there any solution to this deadly problem. Yes of course, there must be. You have to fight like a warrior, a war with your own self, a war for the sake of your present and future, for your parents and beloved ones. What to do in order to conquer your quest. You need to put forth your self esteem and make use of your will power. The more you will strengthen your will power, the more satisfaction you will gain out of this noble fight.

Secondly, you should know what is more important to you, alcohol or something else. Of course alcoholism is not your priority. Now this is the point where you outline your small preferences and future aims that will help you fighting this evil.

Accept the fact that you are in trouble. Accept it that you got into this trap because of your own self. But instead of self pity, that is a curse, quit it at once. If you think that quitting this habit at once can cause some serious damages to your health then you are very much mistaken. Of course, quitting alcoholism will cost you something regarding physical pain but these health issues would be better then losing your precious life forever for nothing. So be honest with yourself, accept the reality, face this challenge, and stick to it until you succeed.

To develop a new repertoire of behaviours after being stuck in the alcoholic loop is not as easy as it sounds. Certainly, it is an uphill task. Most people who try to "quit" make the decision without a clear understanding of the challenge that lies ahead of them.

Be ready for the cruel but temporary outcomes when you quit it. But remember you are developing a healthy relation with yourself by letting yourself know about the importance of your existence. The best way to avoid these temporary moments is going out with your loved ones. You will feel sense of satisfaction by looking at their happy faces. Make yourself busy with books and movies and try seeking spiritual attachment with God. Spirituality is the ultimate solution but again if you are willing to fight back.

WHAT DRIVES ONE SIBLING TO ALCOHOLISM AND THE OTHER TO A PRODUCTIVE LIFE

I come from a middle class family, born and raised in suburbia. As my father always said, you were born with a silver spoon in your mouth, boy. While that is not entirely accurate, the saying does ring true in many aspects of my life. I have never had to fight for anything in my life, I have never had to worry about the next time I would get a meal, and I have never worried about where I would sleep that night. In a certain sense, I am spoiled.

Based on this premise, neither I nor any of my four brothers and two sisters (I know, that's a big family) should fall short of the potential in our lives. We were raised with every opportunity to succeed, and every safety net to catch us if we stumbled or fell. Our parents paid for nearly each and every one of us (with the exception of the eldest brother because he decided to join the army) to attend college and graduate with a Bachelors degree. Therefore, this type of environment should propagate only fruitful individuals.

Working in hospitals and clinics, I have seen what happens to children that are neglected and treated with disdain. It is a sad sight to witness a child falling behind in her development while the mother ignores this and yells at the child, I told you to shut up while I'm talking.' Then the mother calmly brings her attention back to me to finish describing why the employees at the social service office are 'full of a bunch of selfish assholes' for not listening to her situation in order to receive WIC supplements.

With the thought of that mother in your head, it is hard to understand how an individual that is born with a silver spoon in his mouth could slowly dissolve his life in alcohol. He has every opportunity to live a fulfilled life; however, he fights every day to not regress. At this point in time, he is not winning the fight.

Thus, it has become my personal interest to determine what factors predispose an individual to alcoholism, as well as the factors that trap him or her in a state of continual relapse despite the degree of intrinsic motivation that person may have. As I work with my brother through his disease I pick up a gem of knowledge every day about how to help him, myself and anybody else that is affected by alcohol or a loved one of an alcoholic.

MERIT OF USING RESIDENTIAL TREATMENT TO FIGHT ALCOHOL ADDICTION

Alcohol is a part of the life of billions of people. For many, for most of them it is not a concern for their health. But for others it is the basis of a serious disease. Addiction to alcohol can cause the destruction of your marriage, the loss of your job, the breakup of your family and even your premature death. It can be a dangerous and deadly product. And so the millions of people who are in trouble because of alcohol have a simple choice; do they wish to beat their addiction?

Once they decide to try and beat the disease, there are basically two ways they can try to do so. They can seek professional help as a day or out patient, or they can reside in a facility; they can live in.

Now take the option of the day patient. Here the person goes about their normal routine, perhaps going to work, and then at night goes to the clinic or treatment facility and receives whatever they need and is available. This is a sensible and relatively inexpensive way of tackling the alcohol problem. And of course the person is free to attend a support group such as Alcoholics Anonymous.

But what needs to be understood here is that the drinker's environment is often their worst enemy. If they are used to drinking at home and they return to their home after their daily or weekly treatment, they are returning to temptation. They are increasing the chance of failing to beat their disease. So saving money by becoming a day patient may count for little if, back in your comfortable environment, the patient gets back on the drink.

That's why being a residential patient is, in many ways, so much better.

It's not better financially because living in a detox center or rehabilitation facility does not come cheap. But there are many advantages. You get constant access to medical professionals who are trained to work with people who have a problem with alcohol. At the end of each day when your treatment sessions are over, you do not have to find transport in order to go home. You are home. You are living in the center. And this means of course that the temptations you faced when living at home are no longer present. Obviously there will be no alcohol available in the facility and you are not permitted to head into town to find the nearest bar or bottle shop. Your chances of overcoming your addiction to alcohol are far greater if you become an inpatient.

There are often a variety of approaches in overcoming alcohol addiction and centers use a variety of activities. Living in means you have access to all types of treatment and at most times of your stay. And because alcohol can badly affect both the physical and mental aspects of the drinker's life, having a range of medical experts available gives you, the patient in residence, and the best possible form of treatment.

FETAL ALCOHOL AND WHAT DOES IT HAVE TO DO WITH ME?

Fetal Alcohol Spectrum Disorder, (FASD) is not a mental health diagnosis or a medical diagnosis but is an umbrella term used to describe a range of syndromes and disorders that can occur in a child whose mother consumed alcohol during pregnancy. The effects and symptoms vary in severity. Many children share the common effects which include emotional, physical and learning difficulties. The common physical characteristics that can be associated with FASD are facial deformities, growth deficits, heart, liver, kidney defects, vision and hearing problems as well as permanent brain damage. FASD is the only 100% preventable cause of mental retardation and birth defects in the United States and FASD is 100% untreatable. It is estimated that FASD affects 40,000 infants each year. This is more than Spinal Bifida, Down Syndrome and Muscular Dystrophy combined.

Alcohol damages the parts of the brain that gives us memory, self-control, coordinator and judgment. Children with FASD often have difficulties with learning, attention, memory, central nervous system, and problem solving skills that may have lifelong implications. FASD is a permanent condition and affects every aspect of the child's life and the life of their family.

The emotional toll on families cannot be underestimated. For birth parents, acknowledging that their child's mental retardation, birth defects, and/or neurodevelopment disorders are a result of maternal prenatal alcohol consumption is very difficult to face. For adoptive or foster parents, discovering that their child suffers from FASD after years of trying to understand his cognitive and behavioral problems results in feelings of frustration and isolation.

As an adoptive mom I can tell you raising a child with FASD is the hardest but the most rewarding thing I have ever done. Andrew is now 13 years old and is in the seventh grade. He is sweet, generous, loving and very naive. He also has exhibited many of the symptoms associated with FASD since the day we brought him home at 1 week old. He cried all the time! Until he was 3 years old and on medication he never slept for more than 30 minutes at a time, day or night. To say life seemed impossible is actually an understatement. He required constant attention and if I let him out of my sight in another room for one minute he would destroy it. If I was not right beside him when he had a bowel movement in his diaper he would take it off and smear feces all over the walls, carpets and bed. We had to put a lock on our refrigerator because he would climb out of his crib in the middle of the night and dump everything out of the refrigerator smearing it in the carpet, walls, and beds. For years we knew that there were serious problems, but no one could help us. All of the professionals said that his behaviors were out of their expertise. We went from Doctor to Doctor, counselor to counselor and searched everywhere for answers for him and our family. By the age of three, he was thrown out of every daycare in our area, went through at least 30 babysitters, and could not stay in the nursery at Church. He was very violent toward everyone; however most of his rages were taken out on me. He would bite me, hit me and throw things at me. He would put holes in the wall, windows, threw rocks at us, as well as the cars and was basically never happy. When he started school a whole new nightmare started. The fourth day of school he had thrown toys, supplies and destroyed the classroom than ran out of the room causing the teacher to have to leave other students to chase my 4 year old. He was moved to an emotionally disabled class where they had experience with other children like him.

By the time he was 5 he had so many diagnoses I lost count, but none of them actually explained the severity of his behaviors. We had tried 21 different medications and tried at least 4 different kinds of therapy. We started researching the internet and found a few sites about FASD and found that there were several places in the USA that specialized in FASD. Andrew and I packed up, leaving my husband and other two children at home and went in search of a diagnosis. We went to Baltimore, MD and saw a FASD specialist that finally gave him an accurate diagnosis of Fetal Alcohol Syndrome. While we finally had a diagnosis nobody seemed able to help us get his behavior under control and his behavior was getting worse. At that time, he was on 7 medications however none were effective. We went back on the internet searching and learning about FASD and found a "severe" behavior clinic, The Marcus Institute, in Atlanta GA. They observed his behaviors and they immediately asked if we would be open to coming to Atlanta to live for a couple of months so he could attend the clinic. It was their observation that his behaviors were something that would not ever get better without extreme intervention. At this point we had no choice; he was getting bigger, stronger and more destructive every day. After fighting insurance complications, Andrew and I went to Atlanta where he underwent treatment, testing and training for eight weeks.

After two months of hard work the severe behavior clinic was able to decrease his problem behaviors by 96.6% from when we first started the program. The skills we learned are skills we are still using to keep his behavior under control. While we still have bad days, we also now have good days. He is able to stay at school all day now, with the help of a shadow and he is able to play baseball and football with other kids his age and he is happy.

Andrew, as well as most FASD children will never be what others feel is "normal" and that is okay with us because he is now a happy little boy. He is learning to read, and is slowly learning social skills. We had to adjust our expectations as well as learn to think "outside of the box" when we are dealing with him and his problems. We are living a fairly normal life, whatever that is. We are not healed in the traditional sense but we are functioning and making progress. He is now off of 5 of the 7 medications and has really grown physically and emotionally.

Most children with FASD have many issues to face their entire lives. FASD behaviors are treatable but not a curable condition that can be fixed with therapy or medication. There are some children who benefit from certain types of medication, but the medications only address some of the symptoms. Permanent brain damage cannot be fixed or medicated. Creative behavior management works well most of the time. Children with FASD have processing problems and cannot understand cause, effect, or consequences. One of the most important things I have learned from my son is to keep an open mind, a sense of humor, and my faith in God.

ALCOHOL ABUSE AND WORKING OUT - NOT THE BEST MIX

I'm going to put myself out there a little on this one because it hits home for me. I'm not so much coming from the perspective of people that work out then go party on the weekends though I'll touch on that as well. I'm more so coming from the perspective of people who suffer from alcoholism and have a problem with it. With that I could easily tap into substance abuse with this subject but we'll stick to excessive drinking.

Sure, there are those who seem to have more control and these are the ones that may work out during the week and do it up on the weekends, or perhaps just on occasion. I won't go as far as to say that if you do this you'll negate all of your gym efforts (unless it's excessive every weekend, which you fool yourself if you don't think this can quickly turn into a real problem). But it certainly isn't going to push you towards your ultimate goal. Then again, that all depends on how serious you are. For those of us who suffer from chronic abuse this will indeed hold us back from our full potential.

First of all excessive alcohol will lower your testosterone levels. We know that with men testosterone is a key factor in building muscle and burning fat. Alcohol is also considered empty calories which are stored as fat. You also have to consider not only the calories in alcohol but the substances that are often mixed with it. It's clear that alcohol is counterproductive in many ways to building a strong and muscular physique. As if this weren't enough have you ever tried to work out the day after a night of drinking? It's not going to be pretty and you can forget about giving your best efforts. One night of binge drinking can set you back several days, if not an entire week. There's also a long list of health problems that can develop from alcohol abuse.

Sadly enough this is something that many struggle with. I've been there myself. Whether you're into bodybuilding or just love the feeling and effects of intense workouts, we can all agree that this is an extreme sport in its own way. With that being realized it's easy to see that some of us get caught up into other extremes in life. Many of us that workout intense are addicted to working out to some degree, though a healthy addiction. But none the less that personality trait on addiction is there and is often prevalent in our lives.

Those cravings seem to come and go. One thing I've learned that helps is acknowledging this as a true problem and seeing it for what it is. This helps you stay on guard at all times. When you feel those moments of vulnerability coming on you're able to take a step back. It doesn't mean we won't ever fall but it may mean that we fall less often, and when we do, we'll be able to get back up and fight again. We also have to constantly remind ourselves why we do what we do in regards to the gym. It's more than just strength on the outside or attaining a muscular physique. Sure, that's part of it. But it's more so an inner struggle that we're able to conquer day in and day out. We prove something to ourselves every time we tap into this strength that we pull from deep within and push through another day. When we dwell on the very thing that makes us become a better person every day, we then realize we can conqueror this evil, and so we do yet another day.

SEVEN WAYS TO STOP DRUG AND ALCOHOL ABUSE

The problem, the stigma, the black mark that crushes everyone's life - drugs, illegal drugs, over-the-counter drug use, how do we stop it? No one has the perfect answer on how to stop people from using drugs, but there is one way that you can give your children better chances than they might have when it comes to winning the war against drugs. How do I know this - from personal experience, from living life, from growing up in the generation of flower power and the era when drugs were prevalent and widespread throughout the large cities in America. What was one of the things that helped keep me away from drugs when drugs were all around me? If you knew the answer of how to stop your children from using drugs would you use the solution?

Nothing is guaranteed, of course. Everyone is an individual and of course, if one person wants to do drugs and if one person feels they need to do drugs, then that person will abuse drugs. However, there are little things, ordinary things that we can do to guide our children in the better directions in life, and these little things have been proven to work on most children. Here is how you can give your children a head start, a running start in the race against illegal drugs in your society.

Enforce an atmosphere where time is valuable and that valuable time is filled with good events, good projects, and valuable hobbies. Any time that is spent doing good, doing productive projects, being busy being creative is that much less time that any person will spend doing drugs or being hooked on drugs. introduce your children to being creative, to having a hobby, to becoming very interested in bringing good into their lives and you will have given your children an anti-drug asset. If you look at other teens and adults, it is usually the teens and adults that are occupied with LIFE that have no time and have no interest for illegal drug use. So, first priority, get your child or teen interested in a hobby that rocks their world. Let them choose the hobby and that hobby will last them a lifetime.

Teach your children the valuable lesson that God is forever with them, wherever they are, with no matter what they are doing. When children realize that God is with them, right there, at that very moment, then children - when approached by drug dealers -- will just say no. Anyone who believes in God and believes that God is with them in every moment of their lives will be stronger when it comes to fighting against drug use. Faithful believers are generally much stronger, emotionally than people who believe in nothing. The reason for this is because it is common sense that two are stronger than one. So when a child has a strong faith in God, that child is never alone. That child has a Buddy that will help that child fight the urge to join the drug users. That works! That child has someone they can call on in times of temptation and weakness, and most times, that simple solution to life's' problems does work.

Talk to your child about drugs. Give them the information that they need to have in their lives. But most importantly talk to them about drugs even when you think that they are too young to know about drugs. No child is too young to learn about illegal drug use. Your approach in the talk will be different depending on the age of the child. But every single child should be taught about illegal drug use. Besides this talk to them about alcohol abuse.

KNOW that there are sometimes direct links between alcohol abuse and illegal drug use or abuse of prescription drugs. There are times when a child or teen will be very vulnerable to using illegal drugs when normally they would not dream of toughing the product. These times are the times when a child is weak or vulnerable - for example, if a child or teen has abused alcohol or is really drunk. That child will possibly accept drugs if that child is drunk when normally that child had the attitude of "just say no" to drugs. This is how educated children or teens get hooked on drugs when they have, all their life, been anti-drug. So, a clear, present, solid education on alcohol abuse is one of the weapons that you have in your arsenal against illegal drug use and against prescription drug use.

Keep your prescription drugs out of the medicine cabinet and keep them inside a locked box away from children and teens. Every child has a bit of temptation inside of them. It is best to get the drugs out of plain view. The bathroom and the medicine cabinet are private places. Children and teens can look through there and experiment in there and you would never know it happened. Knowledge is your second weapon against drug use. So keep all and any prescriptions locked up and out of the bathroom. Throw out all old prescriptions. You do not need them if they have been sitting for years. They are not valuable to you and if you need them again, you should go to the doctors and get new prescriptions.

Clear your home out. You can have alcohol in your home, just do not have a liquor store inside your home. Do not make your home a storage home for abundant alcohol or prescription, or illegal or legal drugs. This is so important in fighting the drug war. Why have a stock of these items when children and teens are in the house. Children and teens are natural curious people and they are experimenters. There are children and teens who never would have been hooked had the product not been in the home. So do your best. If you need a supply of anything in your home, make it a supply of good reading books, and good music and wonderful creative projects and arts and crafts items.

Do not use illegal drugs yourself. Just say no! When your child or teen sees you abusing drugs, illegal or legal, you are teaching your child how to live. You do not want to teach that lesson. If you think that you can take illegal drugs and not set a bad example, you are mistaken. I know of one family who used pot but forbid the children to use pot because it was illegal. Of course, that child grew and when that child reached a certain age, that child became a full time drug user. That child grew up to be a drug dealer, and wound up in jail and is now currently either in jail or in a half-way house. That child has a lifetime of illegal drug use. That same child who watched his parents smokes "recreational pot". Sometimes your children will not have the strength or resistance that you might have. So do not think that you can take drugs into your home and not promote these drugs to your own children. Do not use illegal drugs and do not abuse alcohol or prescription drugs. Care about your children even if you do not care about yourself. Please save your child's life by not doing anything illegal.

Doing any or all of these things in your home will give your child and your teen strength and possibilities of avoiding illegal drug use and avoiding prescription drug abuse and avoiding alcohol abuse. Try your best to follow the instructions listed above and you will be giving your child and teen a head start in this world. It is worth trying. Yes, there are no guarantees in life. I am not saying that if you do all this that your child or teen will never take drugs. However, I am saying that if you do all these things or most of these things, your child will have better reasons to live, better reasons to enjoy life and your child will have a 85 percent chance of fighting illegal drug use and alcohol abuse than any other person has in their life. Do it. Try it. What do you have to lose? You have nothing to lose and everything to gain. This is your child's life that we are talking about. Wouldn't you do anything to save your child's life? Most people would. Now, in that perspective, all those actions seem like very easy things to do!

So, what makes me an expert on illegal drug abuse? Here is how I come across this gem of information that definitely saves lives. I grew up in a city that was filled with drugs. I could get drugs whenever and wherever I wanted to. Yet, I used the policy of "Just Say No" -long before this project came out to television. That was my motto. I just said no. It is easy to just say no BEFORE you are hooked, before you ever touch an illegal drug. And that is why you begin early. Catch your child's interest before they have a chance to take drugs, and then you have the head start. So, back to the story, most of my friends began taking drugs. (I hung out with a group of friends and little by little, I noticed that they were trying marijuana. The minute I saw that they were using illegal drugs, I ran from my friends and I ran to my "hobby". It was my hobby that saved me from trying drugs and it was my hobby that saved me from being like my friends. That's all it took, one hobby. Instead of becoming introduced to drugs I become fully attentive to my hobby. I am telling you from first hand experience that a hobby gives your child or teen an eighty-five percent chance - better than the average person's chance to stay away from illegal drug use, and other abuses.

Where does faith and belief come in? I am not talking about religion. Religion has never saved anyone from drugs. I am talking about a sincere faith and belief in God and or in the Bible. That is where the strength comes from. And this is your backup plan (which should be your first plan, but everyone is individual). At times when a person is so vulnerable that they are too tired, too weak or too busy or preoccupied to reach for or to think of their hobby, that is where faith comes in. Everyone can pray; everyone can reach out to God. All it takes is a thought. That is why faith is so wonderful. Faith requires no physical effort. So faith fills in where the hobby left off. Even if you are totally exhausted and can not move, you still have the energy left for prayer, a silent prayer or verbal prayer. You can pray.

By using all of the above tools you can possibly safeguard your child and teens from jumping into the world of illegal drugs and alcohol and prescription drug abuse.

So, what was the outcome of my own tools? I grew up with almost everyone around me using illegal drugs. My knowledge let me "leave" the group and run to my hobby. I never even touched a marijuana cigarette. I never took one illegal drug. That is enough proof for me that this system and these tools works. I have many friends who have died from drug use and have many other friends who wound up in rehabs and had miserable lives because they had no hobby to run to and no faith to take over when there was no physical strength to do their hobby. Almost everyone around me, in my circle of friends caved in to peer pressure and caved in to taking illegal drugs. I wonder how many might have stopped short of that if they just had faith or a hobby. None of my friends had a hobby so when marijuana came around, they made marijuana their hobby. Many of them had religion. They had to go to church on Sundays; they had to follow certain man-made religious rules. But none of them had faith in God or faith in themselves. Their faith was in marijuana. Their faith failed them when they needed real faith.

This system works if you dare use it. Yes, yes, yes, I hear you. It is not foolproof, but I guarantee you this. If you use this system, your child will have a better chance than anyone else's child. How do I know? I have proof of it. I just said no! Help your child say no! Bring a system, a plan into your home and into your life. You will be glad that you did.

And deep down inside of every one of us is the challenge, the need to be noticed, to be visible. If there is someone who is invisible in your life today, take a step to bring them into your big picture. You can do it and you will be glad that you did.

I hope you take the advice and I hope that you pass this article around your circle of friends because by doing so, you have the opportunity to save someone's life. And in saving one person's life, you are saving an entire family. People who use drugs ruin lives; they ruin whole families. So please take this step today, and help save your child's life. You will be so glad that you did this.

HELPING THE ALCOHOLIC

To help the alcoholic you love you first must help yourself. You will never be able to help the alcoholic until you help yourself. Alcohol addiction tends to involve everyone the alcoholic is in contact with on some kind of level. Those who are in the path of the alcoholic, usually a spouse, desperately need to know how to emotionally detach from the abuse of the alcoholic. In some cases the mental, emotionally and even physical abuse is so bad that couples must separate.

If the alcoholic begins to get mouthy-calling you names and putting you down, you must leave the room or the house. Remember, the alcoholic is sick and when they drink they are more apt to have emotional outbursts and flared tempers. Don't allow this abuse to sit in your head where it festers and causes emotional problems for yourself.

Let it go in one ear and out the other, literally! You can do this when you understand that part of the sickness of alcoholism is the underlying emotional pain harbored within the alcoholic. Loved ones are usually a scapegoat and temporary outlet for the alcoholic to emotionally unload their demons on, so to speak. I know this first hand because I have been there and done that.

Remember, most of what comes out of the mouth of an alcoholic is the addiction talking. Never take what they say as the gospel truth. When the alcoholic drinks they think they know everything and they may try and get you to believe in the lies and manipulation they are forcing on you. This is how the loved one or enabler becomes sick with the alcoholic. They believe what the alcoholic tells them, at least for a while.

Alcoholics favorite quotes are:

"I am not an alcoholic".

"I can stop drinking anytime."

"I promise I will never drink again"

"You are the one with the problem, not me".

"I only drink to unwind"

"Oh no, I don't have a drinking problem".

"I drink because you treat me bad".

"I'll stop drinking when you stop _____".

Even though none of the above is true the alcoholic may truly believe that what they tell you is true. In their mind, if they are in denial, they may actually believe they can quit just because they say so, but unfortunately addiction doesn't work like that.

One thing that confuses the alcoholic is when you start taking care of yourself, such as reading the bible, praying for them, going to ALANON classes and taking up hobbies. When they see that you are getting emotionally and spiritually well and not letting what they do or say distress you, they will really be miffed.

Walking away or going into another room of the home when the alcoholic starts on a rampage will really annoy them. They expect and even want for you to fight and argue back, scream, yell, cry, or drink with them, not walk away. Don't give them a reaction except for letting them know that you are not going to go down with them into the alcoholism trap.

By all means, let the alcoholic know that you moving on with your life without them. Let them see you becoming emotionally and spiritually well. Nine times out of ten this stirs the conscience within them to start taking responsibility for their problem. They have to want to get sober for themselves and not for you or anyone else.

If you are separated from the alcoholic now because of abuse it is best to make sure the alcoholic has been sober for a full year before they move back into the home. He or she needs to be sober for a while to get used to dealing with life on life's terms. Much healing needs to happen for the alcoholic.

Hopefully after a year of sobriety the alcoholic is not just sober, but has healed emotionally, spiritually and physically from the triggers that made them crave the drink in the first place. Deep inner healing needs to take place within the alcoholic before the alcoholic can actually manage happily without drinking. This is called total sobriety.

Emotional and physical addiction is the areas you will want to look into before total sobriety can be achieved. Know the difference. There is sobriety and then there is total sobriety. Anyone can become sober but not everyone can achieve total sobriety and that's because they still need inner healing, whatever that may be.

Many sober alcoholics continue to go to alcoholics' anonymous years after sobriety. What for? Because it is a crutch they hang onto to keep them from drinking. Other crutches might be another addiction such as sex or food. This is not total sobriety but just a person barely getting by without a drink. That's sad.

God created us to be whole people with the ability to love others and be happy without being a slave to sin, which is what addiction is. We make ourselves become the people we are because of our past and future environments and events and people in our lives. How we manage these circumstances will produce in us the person we become.

If we handle our problems from our own understanding we will walk in err because our own understanding is almost always flawed. We need God in our lives! God does not make alcoholics-we choose what our life is going to be. How we manage life's problems and how we have managed past problems in our life creates a certain lifestyle for us. This lifestyle is made through our choices.

Now this is important, listen well. Just as easily as we became alcoholic or slave to any addiction we can just as easily make ourselves become the child of God that He created us to be. But this is up to the alcoholic-they have to make that choice for themselves. All the people I have known that have truly gotten sober, never craved a drink and became productive happy people in society, God was always at the center of their sobriety.

Stopping Drinking Alcohol - How Important Is It?

Individuals who are suffering from bad case of alcoholism wonder at some point if stopping drinking alcohol is still possible for them. The answer to this is "yes". It is possible for any person, regardless of how severe his or her alcoholism is, to still get back on track and get rid of alcohol. This requires a multi-disciplinary approach that involves professional help, self determination and discipline, lifestyle modification and focus. While it may be difficult at first, there are a lot of innovative as well as alternative approaches that can help and support individuals who want to straighten their lives and overcome alcoholism once and for all.

If you happen to be one of these people who are having a hard time dealing with alcohol problems, or if you know by any chance anybody who is need of help, it is important to recognize the importance of having an alcohol-free life. Stopping drinking alcohol is a very wise step towards appreciating your life and health even more. It can make you realize the importance of your family, wellness, career and future. Moreover, getting rid of alcohol from your system can save you from the potential harm it may cause your health particularly your vital organs such as your liver, stomach and heart among others.

One important approach that can help you in building up your determination to stop drinking is to educate yourself about the harmful side effects of alcohol. Stopping drinking alcohol can actually save your life in so many ways. Thus it is important to understand that drinking excessively and habitually can really lead to serious problems which may be irreversible. It can also impair your vision, judgment and sense of disposition. Furthermore, it no longer comes as a surprise to anybody that a lot of people get into trouble due to uncontrolled drinking. A lot of vehicular accidents and traffic fights happen due to drunk driving. There are also some fatal diseases in which the primary cause is too much alcohol intake such as liver cirrhosis, liver cancer and liver failure.

Stopping drinking alcohol is a mature decision. If you are really determined to get out of the drinking habit, you must not think of it as a short-term goal. Instead, think of it as a long-term goal or a lifestyle that you have to carry on. You must find ways to jumpstart a healthy life like detoxifying your system, eating nutritious and balanced meals, taking a lot of healthy fluids, spending time with your love ones who can provide you the motivation you need, starting new hobbies and engaging in active sports or outdoor activities. There are a lot of things you can do to get your mind of drinking.

If you are determined in stopping drinking alcohol, seeking professional would also be beneficial for you. You can benefit from counselling, support groups and alternative treatment approaches such as meditation, relaxation exercises and hypnosis. It is very important that you know the various options available out there that can help you in getting your life back from alcohol.

TREATMENT FOR ALCOHOL ADDICTION IN 10 EASY STEPS

Most Addictions in general are likely to be really difficult to overcome, as your mind and body will continue craving for whatever you're depriving it of, until you eventually do get a dose of it. Should you occur to be an alcohol addict, or have become addicted to alcohol without really having noticed it, but you most definitely do wish to put a an end to it, then here are 10 great tips for tried and tested treatment for alcohol addiction.

1.) Before even starting, you should make that decision that you truly do want to say goodbye for your addiction. Success in overcoming an dependency only depends on your own personal actions, so if you truly are determined sufficient to make a real start, then you need to!.!

2.) Look for the support of a friend or family member who will be prepared to tend to your needs and listen to your issues although you're overcoming your addiction. Support groups will assist you to stick to your goals and succeed with the treatment of your dependency to alcohol.

3.) Create modifications for your every day routine and lifestyle habits. One of the initial steps which will assist produce the ideal begin in the fight against addiction will probably be by generating drastic changes to your alcohol orientated lifestyle. You will most definitely have to steer clear of any social function that provides alcohol as a refreshment.

4.) Avoid anything that would remind you of drinking alcoholic beverages. Should you smoke, you should also try and quit smoking, which could extremely properly lead you back to the temptation of drinking alcohol again.

5.) You'll require to avoid all of those individuals that influence you with alcohol consumption. Stop hanging out with friends who also abuse alcohol, and this way you will be able to finally forget about alcohol.

6.) Discover methods to manage your daily tension levels. Avoid tension like the plague too as any other issue inside your existence that is often an additional factor to push individuals towards alcohol in the first place, so learn new techniques to overcome tension and other problems in your existence. Exercise, meditation or just going for a quiet vacation would most certainly be a great way to relax.

7.) Seek help from a hypnotherapist. Hypnotherapy is an excellent supplementary therapy for any dependency to alcohol. You can even get a self-hypnosis DVD to assist you to perform hypnosis on your own and keep your thoughts clear of the several tempting thoughts focusing on alcohol consumption.

8.) Attempt cognitive behavioral therapy using the help of a professional therapist. One of the effective methods to beat either alcoholism, general phobias, fears and anxieties, and such addictions is qualified cognitive behavioral therapy. This will assist you to come to terms with your dependency, and will also help you eliminate it as fast as it came into your existence, and also the therapy will also help you discover helpful issue coping abilities to face life's challenges with out resorting back to alcohol.

9.) Carrying out relaxation methods. One of the easiest methods to begin generating some changes in your life is to discover relaxation techniques to assist you to cope using the difficulties of existence and assist you to eliminate any anxiety pains.

10.) Discover new things to assist you to deal using the void left inside your existence. Take on a new sport or interest. Divert your attention to doing productive things that can be enjoyed during your leisure time. A brand new sport, a brand new hobby or even new friends could be the ideal begin to generating a change for the better.

TYPES OF ALCOHOLISM TREATMENTS

Once you've acknowledged that you have a problem with alcohol -- or if you've confronted a loved one about alcoholism -- it's time to start finding ways to treat the problem in an ideal and effective manner. Everyone's body works differently, so there are a few treatment options for alcoholism that may work for you or your family. Here are some suggestions for treatment that will help you decide which method is best for your health.

You will need to consider how long the alcoholism has been going on, the degree of damage that has been done to the body, and the programs and regimens that are available to you in your community. This will help you to make a logical choice that is cost-effective and most likely to work. It may also take more than one method to restore your body and mind back to a healthy state, so make sure that you talk to your doctor regularly to find out how long you should continue one method before switching to something else.

Detoxification is one of the most popular methods of alcoholism treatments, which involves using medicines and even herbal supplements to rid the body of all alcoholic substances. This process can take a few days or weeks, depending on the amount of alcohol in your system. Your physician may also prescribe medication for treating alcoholism, such as disulfiram (Antabus is a popular form of disulfiram) or acamprostate (which will usually come in a brand called Campral). These drugs are used to help prevent relapse and cut down on withdrawal symptoms, while restoring the immune system and other bodily functions. Before you know it, your dependence on alcohol will be diminished.

Counseling, whether alone or with a group, is also a great idea if you're undergoing alcoholism treatment. You should choose the type of therapy that will be most comfortable for you. As you continue attending counseling sessions, you may want to participate in both group and solo therapy. This way you can disclose private thoughts and information to a counselor in confidence, but you can talk about the challenges of living an alcohol-free life with a group of people who can directly relate to your situation. It's also important to be honest during your therapy, no matter what stage you're in. During your sessions, you will discuss the reasons behind your alcoholism and how you feel when you're drinking. You will also discuss which factors made you want to stop drinking and you will have to be truthful to find the root of the problem and avoid falling into alcoholism again. This will help you avoid being fooled into thinking you can fight alcoholism on your own. You need a dependable system of family, friends, counselors, and doctors to ensure you're able to live a healthy and happy life from here on out.

Common Signs of Alcoholism

Someone you love may be an alcoholic, and you don't even know it. But knowing the symptoms of alcoholism, and the warnings signs people with alcoholism exhibit, will go a long way towards helping you get them the help they need.

Here are some of the most common signs of alcoholism:

Irresponsible behavior. An individual with a drinking problem will begin to behave in ways that are a danger to himself and others. Driving while under the influence of alcohol, physical and mental abuse of a spouse or significant other, getting into fights, putting one's career in jeopardy by missing or coming in late to work are all examples of irresponsible behavior brought on by alcoholism.

Health problems. The excessive drinking of an alcoholic can lead to some very serious health problems. The alcoholic may experience fatigue, severe headaches, joint pain, anxiety, loss of weight and other potentially serious health issues. And obviously, the long term health consequences of alcohol abuse are well documented and include liver failure and premature death.

Drinking at all hours of the day. An alcoholic is NOT a social drinker, and as such may begin consuming alcohol first thing in the morning, and then continue on (often drinking alone) throughout the day. This symptom of alcoholism is likely to lead to several forms of self-destruction - most prominent among them, losing one's job.

Increased tolerance to alcohol. The alcoholic will be able to drink a greater-than-normal amount of alcohol without feeling the effects. They will also have a hard time stopping their drinking "binge" once they have begun - a common signal that their tolerance for alcohol has increased.

Blackouts and memory loss. An alcoholic is likely to drink so much that they experience blackouts - periods where they cannot remember anything about their actions. Memory loss due to alcohol abuse is psychologically damaging and highly self-destructive in nature. Although he personally has no memory of it, the alcoholic may say or do things to friends and family, that leave emotional scars that take a great deal of time to heal.

Drinking as a response to stress. An alcoholic drinks when life's problems cause him or her stress. If there's a problem at work or at home, a person with a drinking problem will consume more alcohol (relative to how bad the problem is) in an effort to forget about the issue. Therefore, an alcoholic rarely works to solve problems - and instead drinks to escape them.

Breaking promises. The alcoholic commonly breaks promises he makes to family and friends. These broken promises take the form of missing a child's baseball game or not paying back a loan to a friend. But the most common broken promise that comes from an alcoholic is one he makes to himself: that tomorrow he will stop drinking. That he can get his drinking problem under control without assistance.

Hallucinations. After excessive drinking, many alcoholics will see things that aren't there. These types of hallucinations can cause psychological damage to the alcoholic and lead to bouts of irrational fear and paranoia. Hallucinations are also prevalent among alcoholics going through withdrawal symptoms as they wait for their next drink.

Continue to drink after any of the problems above have occurred. The chief symptom of alcoholism is this dreaded behavior. When a person's health is failing because of alcohol abuse, yet they continue to drink. When they have lost their job and their family because of alcohol, but still pick up that glass. This is the downward spiral of alcoholism that has claimed millions of lives around the world.

If you or someone you love is experiencing any of these symptoms, get them (or yourself) help!

See a professional as soon as possible, before the alcoholic harms another person or does irreparable damage to himself.

INTERRUPTING THE SIGNS OF ALCOHOLISM WILL PROTECT YOU FROM LIVING WITH AN ALCOHOLIC

There are signs of alcoholism you must identify in order to avoid living with an alcoholic. No child ever says "When I grow up I want to be an alcoholic" - or marry one. Yet, too many people today find themselves either having an alcohol abuse addiction or living with an alcoholic. Alcoholism mainly develops gradually and undetected until later stage when life "suddenly" becomes a nightmare. However, there are many signs of alcoholism you can watch for that indicate possible alcohol addiction.

One of the first signs of alcoholism is a high tolerance for alcohol. This can indicate that an individual has a genetic predisposition to alcoholism. If your loved one is capable of drinking until dawn, you may end up living with an alcoholic later in life if early alcoholic intervention does not take place.

In the beginning when most people start drinking, it takes only little to get the effect of the alcohol. Over time, they need more and more alcohol to achieve the same buzz. Even without the genetic disposition, this type of drinker can develop other signs of alcoholism as their alcohol tolerance increases.

If that person has begun drinking alone, drinking secretly or making excuses to drink, you are right to be worried as these, in combination with others, are signs of alcoholism. There is a difference between a reason and an excuse. Reasons are reasonable. An excuse is what the alcoholic will intentionally create to justify drinking. A common excuse from those with an alcohol addiction is "I've had a hard day, I deserve this drink!" but it never stops at one drink as the alcoholic empties one glass - or bottle - after another. There is also "You don't know what my work is like! Drinking helps me deal with my problems!" This leads to the opposite outcome where the alcoholic avoids dealing with his or her life and culminates with you living with an alcoholic.

Other sign of alcoholism includes your loved one has been in trouble for an alcohol-related crime yet continues to drink. According to many treatment centers and mental health experts, this is one of the classic signs of alcoholism. Drinking and driving is one of the most common legal struggles that alcoholics get involved in.

You may be living with an alcoholic if your loved one has an inability to moderate or stop drinking. Perhaps the person have genuinely intended to stop drinking for periods of time in the past but just could not stay away from the alcohol. Or, when one glass leads to another and then a few empty bottles later, it may be followed by violent episodes... yet another of many signs of alcoholism. If you, or your children, are victims of violence, it is critical that you protect yourself (and the children) and leave until it is safe to return!

If you observe these various signs of alcoholism in your loved one, you are right to be concerned and you do need to take action now to avoid ending up living with an alcoholic. Get to know the other signs of alcoholism and learn more about how to help yourself when living with an alcoholic so you can change the situation before it becomes much worse.

Intercepting the signs of alcoholism in their early stages of appearance protects you from ending up living with an alcoholic later on in your life. No matter how advanced the situation is you must take action now. If you treat it as if you already are living with an alcoholic you will have huge advantage and be very effective in dealing with any signs of alcoholism in your home.

SELF-RECOVERY FROM ADDICTION: TAKING RESPONSIBILITY FOR YOUR LIFE

I've had several coaching clients come to me who, while they wanted to move forward in life, were actually stuck in a self-destructive addiction. Of course, I cannot directly confront them about their addictions, as they had to open up to me that it was part of the problem that was keeping them in the same rut in which they found themselves day-after-day. As we worked together to make plans and open doors, the addiction was left open for them to examine and realize that they needed to overcome the situation, and cut loose that anchor to move forward to a fulfilling life.

I'm not speaking of any particular addiction, as we all have one or two in our lives. However, for sake of discussion, the primary addictions that people fall to when they find that their lives are faltering are alcohol and drugs. Of course, these usually come into play once their addictions to depression and negative situations overtake their lives and they feel as though they have no where left to turn. But, as we peel away the negative situations and tend to the depression through medical assistance, they are better able to accept that now they must eliminate the substance addiction.

• Abstinence or Control

Many commercials on television promote "responsible drinking". What exactly is "responsible drinking"? It is a relative view that places you to judge how much is enough. Yet, after your first drink, your judgment is impaired. As I've heard from many people, "one is too much and 12 are not enough." The best way to manage yourself responsibly is simply not to do it at all --- abstain.

• Disease or Responsibility

The idea of addictions being a disease creates an uneasy feeling for me in that, for the most part, it is a choice and a responsibility as opposed to an illness. While I do agree that certain physical illnesses can cause people to turn to substance abuse, the abuse and addiction in and of itself are resulting actions and not diseases. It does seem that the disease concept has become popular because it is the nature of addicted people to dignify their conduct. The disease concept conceals the actual reason people abuse various substances while it discourages initiative and responsibility.

• Involuntary Addiction

This area of "involuntary addiction" is the center of much controversy. Many people are addicted to medications at the hands of medical practitioners who do not monitor their patients, but instead simply ensure that their prescriptions maintain a certain response. Of course, many people do require long-term care; however, others only require assistance through medication for a short time.

One example is that of a woman I worked with some years ago who was terribly addicted to Valium, Paxil, and Prozac. She wanted to get off of everything. Of course, I could not counsel her on the medical aspects of her situation, but I did refer her to a medical acquaintance who could assist her. In the end, after six years of involuntary addiction, it took her two years to get back on her feet and lead a productive life. We did work through some situations to angle her life toward her new Vision, but it was her choice to alleviate herself of the medication and "give life a try." In essence, we were able to replace her physical addiction with a mental and emotional addiction --- a direction in life.

• How did I become addicted?

Addiction is a natural function of the human body, based entirely upon the "pleasure principle" --- the tendency to seek pleasure and avoid pain. Addictive substances have the ability to disrupt the motivational hierarchy of needs by displacing other motives in life. They can also desensitize the ability of other, natural rewards to motivate behavior. The addict usually places substance use as their top priority, while losing interest in life's other rewards. This desire to experience the effects of the addictive substance combined with the lack of interest in natural rewards is classified as a "loss of control." Essentially, the normal controls on the individual's life have lost their significance and behavior focuses on the acquisition and use of the addictive substance.

It's interesting to note that we can become addicted to situations as well as substances. For instance, some abused women come to feel a certain way about themselves in abusive situations. To ensure that this feeling remains, they seek out relationships that compound their feelings. Destructive indeed, but one that they feel is necessary.

• How can I tell if I am addicted?

Determining addiction is complex in that it is based on many different signs for different types of addictions. But, the one definite, yet simplistic, indicator is that you keep going back even after you know that you don't want to do it again.

Those nights that you lay in bed with a massive hangover even after you swore that you'd never do it again. The morning you wake up and have no idea what you did the night before, again. The bruises and black eyes that you have from the fight with your mate, yet you return. Again, the simplest indicator is that you "keep coming back."

More complex indicators are physical and emotional changes as well as affects on your social presentation and associations. For instance, massive weight change, the "need" to have it or do it again, anger, loss of sleep, health problems, avoidance by certain social associations, or even being banned from establishments are important indicators.

• How can I achieve recovery?

Recovery is your choice. You must first choose to acknowledge its existence and then you must choose to do something about it. Acknowledge that you are not a victim and take the responsibility that you chose to enter into the addiction. By doing so, you are taking control to be able to take responsibility for choosing to not be addicted any longer.

Abstinence is the first step to recovery. Immediately stop what you're doing, whether it is through counseling, medical assistance, or simply ceasing your addictive actions. Of course, it is easier said than done.

One thing that we do in my coaching sessions is, once a client seeks assistance from qualified medical professionals, we immediately begin to replace the addictive situation with something else that is of benefit. For instance, many of those clients who are addicted to some substance or situation are because they don't know what else to do or need to move in a direction away from a current situation. With nothing else in life, they drink, use drugs, or continually place themselves back into situations that are consistent and provide the "comfort zones" that keep them in an arena that feels safe.

• A replacement addiction?

While replacing one addiction with another does not sound appealing, indeed, it is a path that is essential to the success of recovery. For instance, while I may not agree with support groups, many people find them useful and a necessary part of life. Indeed, while these are a replacement addiction for the other addiction, they are not as harmful as the addiction that they replace. At the very least, such support groups are a reasonable replacement of the addiction until the person is strong enough to stand up against their previous addictions.

For many of my clients, they have found that by defining a plan for their life, instead of meandering to the point of getting lost and addicted to something else that is harmful, they are better able to cope with their recovery. With help from their medical professional, along with a life plan, they can remain focused and busy while working toward their Vision. In the process, their values change to the point that they no longer require a substance to give them the necessary feelings that they pursue.

One example was a young man whose father committed suicide. It threw him into a cycling depression where, at one moment he was fine and, over a period of months, he would be depressed again and have to work to recover from the depression. In the process, he turned to a serious alcohol addiction, which nearly disrupted his entire life. After focusing on the core depression and working with his doctor to stabilize his emotions, we worked together to find a way to piece together a new life. Indeed, with the loss of a family member, life does change, yet he was unable to cope with this change as he was caught in the life he had prior to the loss.

Realize that the addiction can take on a mind of its own and will eventually do anything to ensure that it gets what it wants. It can begin to define you. However, it is essential to turn that hunger into something else with a different focus and desire. That is the core success of recovery.

• What's next?

Inside of every addicted individual is the original person who was full of wonder and excitement about the possibilities that lay ahead. Somewhere along the way, this person became lost and fell prey to the pleasures of their addiction. They instinctively decided that the greatest pleasures that life comes from the use of a substance and they reordered their life to accommodate this new desire at all costs --- this is the destructive point of addiction. It is here that they must make a choice and engage in a fight for survival.

There are a number of pitfalls common to self-recovery from addiction. Those who want to help you, but were never addicted themselves, have little to share on the subject, as their experience and beliefs are based on information provided by equally misinformed books and experts. Additionally, our society sees addiction as a noble affliction and denies that self-recovery is possible. As a result, society does not reward, and sometimes punishes, people who accept personal responsibility for their addictions and their recovery.

Realize that, if your environment has changed because of your addiction, all is not lost. If your family left or you lost your job or even if you lost some aspect of your life, the final decision that you make to move on with your life is the one that matters the most above all. You still have yourself and, in the long run, that is truly all that matters. Spend some time with your

real self, as you might be surprised at the hero
you just found!

ALCOHOL TREATMENT IS NOW VERY POSSIBLE

It is quite an obvious fact that there are many individuals indulging in alcohol abuse. Many of them have become very addicted that they cannot do without taking in doses of alcoholic drinks and related substances. All over the world, beginning with the US, many people are endangering their lives on daily basis as they dabble into alcohol. Many are now dependent on alcohol as a way of escape from the real world.

People who get intoxicated with alcohol end up disgracing themselves at the slightest provocation. They are usually known to be very restless whenever they can't find their favorite alcoholic drink or substance. Such individuals usually purchase enough alcoholic elements daily for their use. However, there are people who really want to break way from it. Other peoples especially a wife whose husband is a heavy drinker and hard drug lover could do a lot to help her addicted man if he is actually into the habit.

Currently, Alcohol Treatment is now very possible. This begins with the assistance of the treatment center where the addict is having his or her treatment. The Alcohol Treatment is usually handled the way most addictions are handled. There are various treatment programs involved in the handling process. These include: in-patient treatment plan, out-patient treatment plan, withdrawal plan and many more.

The process of Alcohol Treatment commences when the addict is admitted for treatment in a rehab center where such cases are handled. Usually the medical professional subjects the addicts to various tests in order to determine the level of alcoholic addiction in their lives. If the alcohol level has gone very far, the person is therefore hospitalized. Other treatment processes follow suit.

On the other hand, if the patient's case is still very minimal, he or she is placed under out-patient plan. With such a wonderful plan, the addict is sure to break loose from the grips of alcohol as he or she comes from home to take the treatment.

Alcohol Treatment also involves a withdrawal process. This is actually not all that easy as most alcohol addicts have made the stuff their second nature. The withdrawal process is never very rosy on the part of the addicts. It is always a very difficult process that may generate after-effects such as sever headache, stomach pain, fever, nausea and many more. However, one must understand that there is always a price to pay in order to break loose from the grips of alcohol. It is better to pay the price and regain your freedom than to just ignore it and watch your life ebb away gradually.

In the final analysis, Alcohol Treatment indeed is not a joke when you want to go for it. There is nothing like 'having fun' in it. It is a pure medical approach aimed at helping the addicts come out of the habit and begin to live normal alcohol-free life. The treatment therefore calls for adequate preparedness and determination on the part of the addicts.

Alcohol is the intoxicating agent in fermented drinks. Typically, it is a colorless liquid substance usually produced by the fermentation of sugar or starch and used in the manufacturing of various beers and other drinks.

All over the world, there are many drinks being manufactured with alcohol. A good number of them do come with high concentration while others do come with less. In the world today, many people are into the habit of daily consumption of alcoholic drinks. Taking alcohol is not a problem or an illegal stuff, but the issue of getting intoxicated is where the problem lies. Many people are getting addicted to alcohol and this does not augur well with their well being.

The abuse of alcohol and its addiction has indeed left many people miserable. The constant intake of alcohol is never for the good of the body tissues and other important parts making the body sound and healthy. It is well known fact that alcohol is very dangerous to health especially to the nervous system of man. Getting intoxicated with alcohol is capable of leading to mental disorder, hallucination, brain damage and other forms of disorders. Many times it leads to alteration of the chemical process of the body and in extreme cases; it can lead to the damage of the sperm production in men.

The panacea to the above situation is simply through Alcohol Treatment. This is indeed the process of getting alcohol addicts free from the grips of the intoxicating agent. Many people who engage in incessant intake of alcohol find it difficult to miss it even for a day. For so many alcohol addicts, life is meaningless without alcohol and a day is not well spent without the gulping of various kinds of alcoholic drinks.

Indeed, Alcohol Treatment is not a day's job. It takes much time depending on the seriousness and response of the addict involved. The treatment process begins with the arrival of the addict into any of the reliable addiction treatment centers or Alcohol rehab centers. In such establishments, there are trained medical professionals already on ground to deal with the issue.

Addicts whose situations have gone too far beyond the danger zone are normally hospitalized and put under the in-patient treatment program. In such treatment plan, detoxification is introduced. This is the process of removing all the alcoholic drinks from the reach of the addict. The process of withdrawal comes with bodily reactions such as: stomach pain, fever, headache and nausea but with time the patient gets over them.

Again, Alcohol Treatment also involves the used of counseling sessions where cognitive therapeutic methods are also engaged in discovering the causes of the addiction. Useful step-by-step programs geared towards arresting the addiction habit is also shown to the addict.

Finally, the Alcohol Treatment plan also involves after-care programs such as getting involved with Alcoholics Anonymous which is a fellowship of former alcoholic addicts who are now free but are also engaged in helping others regain their freedom from alcohol.

WHEN ALCOHOL ABUSE CHANGES TO ALCOHOLISM

Changing a Person's Drinking Behavior

Thousands of books and articles have been written and countless research studies have been undertaken regarding alcoholism. In spite of this, the one finding that has apparently failed to reverberate throughout the alcohol abuse and alcoholism academic and medical communities is the emphasis on the fact that alcohol addiction has its roots in alcohol abuse. While this fact has many ramifications, perhaps the key upshot of this fact is that millions of non-alcoholic individuals in our society and throughout the world who engage in abusive drinking can address their drinking consumption and make healthy and positive changes in their drinking behavior before they become alcohol dependent.

One school of thought sees alcohol abuse in the following way: alcohol abuse takes place whenever an individual's drinking causes a problem in any aspect of his or her life.

The area of a person's life where alcohol abuse commonly leads to problems includes the following:

• relationships

• employment

• school

• finances

• health

• the law (for instance, a DUI).

The Need for Positive and Healthy Change

Now that we are aware of the problems that are usually associated with alcohol abuse, it can be seen that in order to overcome these difficulties and issues it is important for the alcohol abuser to look in the mirror and honestly ask himself or herself if alcohol is causing a problem in any facet of his or her life.

As an additional component in the quest for healthy and positive change, problem drinkers need to understand that continued, repetitive, and heavy drinking can and does turn into alcohol addiction. Stated differently, millions of non-alcoholics in our society who have a drinking problem will, at some point in their lives, experience a transition from alcohol abuse to alcohol dependency. When this happens, it must be emphasized, the person will no longer simply be an alcohol abuser. Indeed, at this point, the person will be an alcohol abuser and an alcoholic.

SIGNS OF ALCOHOL ADDICTION

How can a person tell if he or she is alcohol dependent? First, the experience of alcohol withdrawal symptoms when an individual suddenly stops drinking is one sign that alcoholism has reared its ugly head.

Second, repetitive and out-of-control drinking behavior is another indication that a person has become an alcoholic. What this usually means is that after consuming the first drink, the individual lacks control over stopping his or her drinking and therefore continues to drink until he or she becomes inebriated.

Alcohol Addiction Has Its Roots in Alcohol Abuse

Perhaps the key in all of this is the following: most, if not all instances of alcohol addiction get their start from alcohol abuse. Stated another way, it is highly unlikely that a non-drinker will become alcohol dependent simply by having one drink or that a non-drinker will become an alcoholic by getting drunk once. Indeed, alcoholism does not result from infrequent and sporadic drinking but rather from continuous, excessive, and repeated drinking. The point: alcoholism doesn't take place in a vacuum. In short, the roots of alcoholism are found in alcohol abuse.

Knowing this and letting this "fact" influence an individual's drinking behavior in a positive and healthy manner is perhaps the single most important health-related bit of information that a problem drinker can learn and implement in his or her life.

Why is this so important? Research shows that alcoholics are masters of denial, deception, dishonesty, and manipulation and often blame their alcohol-related problems on situations and people outside themselves. Alcoholics also exhibit out-of-control and irresponsible drinking behavior. Not only this, but most alcoholics will lie, cheat, and steal in order to get their next drink. Why would an alcohol abuser who is not yet an alcoholic want to face such a dreary and destructive set of circumstances?

The Mixed Messages in our Society About Drinking Alcohol

An Issue of Mixed Messages

How can something as prevalent, accepted, and accessible in our society as drinking alcohol be so harmful, unhealthy, AND illegal when consumed at or slightly above moderate intake levels? The simple asking of this question immediately uncovers a number of issues, one of which is the mixed messages that exist in our society about drinking alcohol.

The Accessibility
and Acceptability of Alcohol

On the one hand, consider the thousands upon thousands of bars and taverns in the United States. Now add to this list the restaurants, night clubs, sporting events, festivals, state fairs, hotels, casinos, carnivals, etc. where alcoholic beverages are regularly served. Moreover, add the grocery stores, liquor stores, beverage stores, the Convenient Food Marts, the 7/11 stores, and the state stores where an adult can legally purchase as many bottles, cans, and/or cases of alcoholic beverages as he or she desires.

Is Drinking Alcohol Cool?

Not only is alcohol extremely accessible in our society but there are also a number of factors that reinforce the idea that drinking alcohol is "cool." For instance, consider beer advertisements and commercials on TV. Indeed, it can be argued that some of the most memorable, funniest, and "best" commercials and advertisements on TV have been those that were associated with drinking beer. To push the point further, why would beer manufacturers spend millions of dollars for a commercial during the Super Bowl if this expenditure did not lead to more sales? From a slightly different perspective, consider professional athletes and movie stars who, by their actions and advertisements, reinforce the idea that drinking alcohol is "cool."

Religious Rituals and Cultural Traditions

When religious rituals that make use of alcohol, cultural traditions that encourage drinking alcohol, special events and holidays that are associated with drinking alcohol, and the increasing popularity of adding alcohol to food for enhanced flavor--when all of these are factored into the equation, it becomes obvious that alcohol is deeply ingrained in our society. The point: when people are surrounded with alcohol and bombarded by events, traditions, holidays, and advertisements that are alcohol-related, it becomes part of their socialization process that in turn makes it easier to simply accept that they should drink alcohol if they are to "fit in" and become members of our society.

Alcohol Abuse and Drinking While Driving

If the prevalence, acceptability, and accessibility of alcohol represent the one side of the coin regarding the mixed messages in our society, then the dangerousness, unhealthiness and illegality represents the other. Indeed, consider the numerous negative and harmful messages and statistics associated with alcohol abuse and drinking while driving that we have heard from the medical community, federal government, police, and politicians, organizations such as MADD, and school and college administrators.

Mixed Messages and Their Consequences

When something like alcohol use is so intimately ingrained in the fabric of our society, it becomes extremely difficult to significantly alter its use and abuse in a comprehensive and beneficial manner. I assert that one of the consequences of the mixed messages about alcohol use and abuse in our society it that it becomes extremely difficult for many individuals, especially our youth, to realistically see the destructive, unhealthy, and sometimes fatal aspects of alcohol abuse.

The Influence of the Judicial System

Unfortunately, the judicial system and the ways in which it has dealt with alcohol-related offenses is another example of the mixed messages in our society about alcohol. For instance, until very recently, people who have received multiple DUIs have, in many instances, simply received a "slap on the wrist" for their alcohol-related behavior.

Fortunately, some states are becoming more reality and accountability-based and are making it a felony when a person receives his or her 4th DUI within a ten-year period. In Minnesota, for instance, this sentence includes three years in prison and a fine of not less than $14,000.00.

INCARCERATION AND TREATMENT

Sending people to jail for alcohol-related offenses, however, is not a viable "solution" unless the person receives help for his or her alcohol problem while incarcerated. True, the offending person is "off the streets" while incarcerated. When the jail or prison sentence is completed, however, a person who has received alcoholism treatment while incarcerated is more likely to become a responsible person who doesn't continue to drink while driving and less likely to become a repeat offender.

Responsible Behavior

I am not necessarily disagreeing with those who preach "responsible behavior" regarding drinking. The bottom line, however, is one's definition of "responsible behavior." Let me explain. Let's say that I have a lake that is used for swimming and that for whatever reason, hundreds of snapping turtles have populated this lake. Some people may say that "responsible behavior" in this example consists of warning all swimmers about the turtles and telling them to "be careful" while swimming. Others with a different point of view, however, might say that "responsible behavior" in this instance means warning the swimmers about the turtles, telling them to be careful while swimming, AND, at the same time, significantly reducing the turtle population so that there is less chance that the swimmers will get bit.

What Can Be Done?

If our society is more enlightened and more aware of the health hazards, fatalities, and destructive consequences of alcohol abuse and alcoholism, then why don't we practice "responsible behavior" and make alcohol less available, less advertised, less glamorized, and less "cool" while at the same time increasing the advertisements, commercials, and public service messages that emphasize healthy and safe alcohol-free activities and lifestyles?

Help For The Alcoholic

Question: If an alcoholic is unwilling to get help, what can you do about it?

Alcoholics don't respond very well to advice, suggestions, or threats. One would imagine that under these circumstances an alcoholic is doomed to oblivion. You must realize the alcoholic is desperate to get more and more alcohol, and he or she may lie, cheat and steal in order to do so.

Very simply, an alcoholic is a person whose life is controlled by alcohol. They are sick.

Question: If the alcoholic is sick why doesn't he or she just go to the hospital?

Because in the early stages of alcoholism, the alcoholic does not appear sick, in pain, or visibly abnormal. Alcoholics do not comprehend that they are about to become a very sick person, and neither do the people around them.

By the time an alcoholic is in the late stage, he or she is often irrational, deluded, and unable to understand what has happened. The alcoholic is simply not aware of what is going on in his or her body and is in a complete state of denial.

Being an alcoholic is not a curse. The alcoholic is a sick person and should be treated as one. Alcoholics are born with a hereditary, genetic predisposition to addiction having to do with brain chemistry. Alcoholics need to ingest alcohol before the addiction takes hold. Alcoholism is a progressive disease, and without treatment it only gets worse.

If an alcoholic is unwilling to seek help, is there any way to get them into treatment?

Sure the courts force alcoholics into treatment all the time. Rehab centers are overflowing with people who don't want to be there. The real question is, will forcing an alcoholic into treatment guarantee recovery? The answer is no.

A perfect example is the alcoholic with multiple DUI arrests. These folks have all been through one or more alcohol treatment programs. Why didn't any of them stick? The answer is the alcoholic refused to admit to themselves they have a problem.

No alcoholic is hopeless. If you're trying to get an alcoholic sober, learn to accept the fact that the alcoholic is sick, from an illness he cannot control, and neither can you. The alcoholic is addicted and an addict cannot stop on their own volition.

The first step in treating the alcoholic is the detoxification stage. The alcoholic must truly want to stop drinking or detoxification becomes a temporary solution. The biggest symptom to overcome for an alcoholic is their denial of having a drinking problem. An alcoholic is "someone who could be helped and is worth helping only if they decide not to drink.

Once an alcoholic is in treatment, they more than likely will be asked to start attending Alcoholics Anonymous (AA) meetings, usually daily. It is not easy to know when or if an alcoholic is "ready" for (AA). You can't make the decision for them. People bounce in and out of (AA) all the time.

The right alcohol recovery program depends upon the severity and nature of the alcoholic and most importantly their personal level of commitment and motivation. A big part of getting the alcoholic into treatment, is overcoming the hurdle they face of actually going to treatment.

Many of the hurdles are self-imposed, yet like fortified brick walls - to the alcoholic they are impassible. The walls are constructed from fear, shame, embarrassment, and denial. The uncertainty of what they must face is enough to trigger enough stress that they simply refuse to go.

It may never be completely understood what causes alcoholism, and (AA) is only one of many recognized treatments for alcoholism. The difference is its track record for success. More than 700,000 Americans receive alcoholism treatment of one kind or another on any given day. Alcoholics Anonymous (AA) is one of the best treatment options for a recovering alcoholic.

Overcoming denial and enabling is often the first step to successful recovery for the alcoholic. Treatment only works if the alcoholic wants it. Forcing a treatment program on an alcoholic does not work. If an alcoholic is going to get anything positive out of an alcohol treatment program, they must be a willing participant.

The (AA) membership knows the routine as far as the alcoholic is concerned. They are all recovering alcoholics too. They supply the means, knowledge, and opportunity. It's up to the alcoholic to take action. It's part of the reason why (AA) is so effective. Very simply, they understand the alcoholic is a person whose life is controlled by alcohol.

Nagging the alcoholic is not the answer to successful recovery. Or is it an effective method to get an alcoholic to stop drinking. The choice must be made by the alcoholic.

Admitting you're an alcoholic is not a requirement for membership to (AA), it is however, the #1 requirement to your recovery. Don't Drink Today - and get involved. Listen to a speaker. Hear their story. In many cases you'll find it's not all that different from yours.

If you don't like the first meeting you attend, go to a different one. It's not like they're difficult to find. Eventually you will find a meeting you like, with people who care and are will help you through the recovery process.

PARENTS - IF YOU LOVE YOUR KIDS CHOOSE NOT TO DRINK ALCOHOL

A WISE DECISION!

Why would a parent, who may enjoy drinking alcohol, choose not to drink?

They know tragic consequences may be in their children's future, if they drink alcohol and their children follow their example.

Good parents refuse to encourage, enable or model alcohol that could potentially kill their child. They know a double standard does not work! Telling your child not to drink alcohol, when you are drinking, doesn't work! Responsible parents are aware that drunk driving, alcoholism, future drug use, are a small part of what can happen after a child takes it's first drink. Parents who really love their children are willing to give up something they may enjoy themselves for the health and safety of their children.

I believe mothers have the greatest responsibility to their children in this area, because they set the tone of the home! For responsible parents, it is not a big sacrifice to make the choice not to drink alcohol.

A study was done on the brains of young people and the finding was that young brains do not fully develop until they are age twenty-five. Young people need the adults in their life to be good examples. They need parents to direct them and help them make good decisions. The sad fact is that many parents are bad examples and by the time a young person figures life out, they are following the same path as their parents.

If you are questioning this idea of parents abstaining, think of this! How would you feel if your child died in an alcoholic stupor because they just wanted to be like you? If you don't want them to drink alcohol, you must not drink yourself.

There is a movement gaining great popularity today, similar to the anti-smoking campaign, which had great success. This movement is called "Reducing Underage Drinking". It is the result of Congress requesting the National Research Council and the Institute of Medicine to review the evidence on various programs aimed at underage drinking and to recommend a strategy to reduce and prevent it.

The conclusion of the study is simply: Alcohol use by young people is dangerous, not only because of the risks associated with acute impairment, but also because of the threat to their long-term development and well-being.

I recently attended a national conference for this movement and was impressed with all the enthusiasm and excitement generated in teaching our young people not to drink alcohol, until they are twenty-one years old. Organizations from all over the United States gathered to share what they know and their successes. Great strides are being made and young people are really being educated in the dangers of drinking alcohol.

I am very thankful for all that is being done and commend all involved for their dedication and desire to save our young people.

Unfortunately, my only complaint is the lack of an abstinence message in their campaign. They are not making it loud and clear, to young people, that they have the choice not to drink alcohol at all, whatever their age. They are not being taught, "Abstinence is the better choice!" They are only teaching young people not to drink alcohol until they are twenty-one years old. They must believe something magical happens when they attain the age of twenty-one. If they only choose to drink then, there will be no consequences.

WHY DO I BELIEVE ABSTINENCE A BETTER CHOICE?

Once again from the study: 1/3 of youth traffic fatalities involve alcohol. Underage alcohol use is also associated with violence, suicide, educational failure, and other problem behaviors. All of these problems are magnified by early onset of teen drinking: the younger the drinker, the worse the problem. Moreover, frequent heavy drinking by young adolescents can lead to mild brain damage. A young person who begins drinking as a young teen is four times more likely to develop alcohol dependence than someone who waits until adulthood to use alcohol. Almost 14 million Americans abuse alcohol or have developed alcoholism.

My argument for encouraging parents to choose not to drink alcohol is personal, but is backed up by the study. It says that the patterns and consequences of youthful drinking are closely related to the overall extent and patterns of drinking in the society, and they are affected by the same factors that affect the patterns of adult consumption. From this standpoint, it is possible that the most effective way to reduce the extent and adverse consequences of youthful drinking would be to reduce the extent and consequences of adult drinking. It is clear, however that Congress intended for the committee to focus on youth drinking, rather than developing a strategy targeting adult drinking. This is what the committee has done.

The study recognizes that the best way to help our young people to choose not to drink alcohol is to teach adults not to drink alcohol! It worked with tobacco and I believe it can work with alcohol too! Unfortunately that is not yet their focus.

WHY DO I THINK PARENTS SHOULD CHOOSE NOT TO DRINK ALCOHOL?

1. Modeling or example is the best teacher.

2. A double standard doesn't work.

3. Telling a child they should not drink until they are twenty-one is a temporary and potentially devastating solution which teaches them that drinking alcohol is ok. What happens, when they become twenty-one, and they choose to drink and end up destroying their life anyway? The first drink can be the beginning of alcoholism. Fifty percent of those who have alcoholics in their family can become alcoholic. It can also lead to a DUI, at any age, as well as all of the other violent crimes committed while people are drunk.

4. Why teaching our kids to only drink in moderation is a bad choice! Because moderation teaches, "It's OK to drink alcohol." There is no safety in teaching moderation. The only safety is in teaching abstinence. Besides, if you are trying to save your kids from the damage alcohol can do and you drink in moderation you are supporting the alcohol industry by giving them money for their products. Aren't you enabling the alcohol industry to continue their mission to make money, so they can continue to destroy our kids, and families?

There is also another common argument. It is thought; if children are taught to drink at home they will be more responsible. This may be true in some cases but in European countries where this is done, the study reports that these countries are no better off than the United States in terms of the harmful consequences of youth's drinking. Besides underage drinking is a crime and if you encourage your child to drink alcohol you are breaking the law!

Many churches have taught moderation and are now paying a price. They have alcohol problems in their congregations. Some of them have an anti-drinking campaign, themselves.

5. As parents, we need to teach our children to naturally and fully use the abilities, gifts and talents they have been blessed with and encourage them to reach their life's purpose and potential. How can they do that if they use a temporary substance to handle their life or avoid growth? If they think they need a drink of alcohol to have fun, handle a problem or escape from a situation, they will never discover their own capabilities. They will never develop the skills needed to enjoy life to the fullest. Kids need to see adults who do fully live their lives without the crutch of alcohol. They need to understand that life is fulfilling, enjoyable and successful without alcohol.

We love our children and we want to provide for them a healthy life style, which they can enjoy, their whole life. We want to do everything we can, as parents; to be sure they have the opportunity to fully live their lives. We want to keep them safe and in good health. ****Good parents set good examples for their kids****

6. Mothers, who drink alcohol, during pregnancy, may give birth to babies with fetal alcohol syndrome (FAS) or fetal alcohol effects (FAE). Children with FAS may have mental retardation, facial and limb irregularities, heart defects, behavioral problems, shorter height, and lower birth weight.

Finally, choosing not to drink alcohol is a choice parents can make for the success and happiness of their kids and for themselves. If our kids mess up their lives because they choose to drink alcohol, you can be sure your life will be messed up too!

Why do I say this? None of us are immune from the ravages of alcohol abuse. Alcohol has affected my family too. My grandfather and father were alcoholic and each died at the age of 57 after devastating our lives when they got drunk. When I was a teenager I began to drink alcohol but thankfully chose to quit when I had kids. My husband has also stopped. We were not alcoholic but realized abstinence was a better choice for the sake of our kids and the results have been wonderful. In our personal family we do not have tragic alcohol stories about our children.

Unfortunately my extended family has not been as fortunate. Some family member parents chose not to quit drinking alcohol and others chose to quite too late. Some of our younger generation live the consequences of being in jail, are alcoholic and or are addicted to drugs.

None of us have a guarantee that our children will follow our good example. Each child is given the gift of choice, but we can rest assured, if they choose to go down a negative path, we did not contribute to it and by our good example we offer them a better path to return to. In the Bible it says: Teach a child in the way he should go and when he is old he will not depart from it.

From my personal experience, I can testify that choosing not to drink alcohol has brought good consequences to my family. "It is in the home that we form our attitudes." I encourage all parents to choose abstinence. It is one of the greatest gifts you will give to your kids.

THE TOP 5 MISTAKES FAMILIES OF ALCOHOLICS AND ADDICTS MAKE

See if any of these situations are familiar to you.

He didn't like the recovery / rehab approach but we told him he had to do it as it was the only thing available that we knew of

We've given him chances, all our money to bail him out, lawyers, paid medical bills -- why should we now pay for rehab?

We are hoping and waiting for him / her to hit bottom -- they have to decide to change on their own

We are giving them another chance, we've forgiven them so many times; hoping this time it will be different

We're expecting meetings, medications or more motivation will turn their lives around, we can only hope something will work

Making the above mistakes don't work despite people being told these methods should work or are the only or best way to handle an addict. Families committing these errors have had their loved ones continue to ruin their lives despite hospitals, jails, courts, short rehab programs. Still the addict reverts back to using.

Why do they continue to make the same mistakes? People follow advice from friends or groups, not knowing there could be better ways to do things. If it's not working for you, it's not working.

THE 5 TOP WAYS TO HELP AN ADDICT OR ALCOHOLIC WITHOUT ENABLING THEIR ADDICTION

Research all options before sending to rehab and pick one that fits the person

Bailing someone out for acting irresponsibly is a major mistake. This does not help them recover, but instead shows them someone else takes responsibility / accountability for their actions. Rehab is the ONLY investment you should be making to rehabilitate the individual

Don't wait for another bottom. Instead, learn everything you can about intervention, consider a pro and coordinate a family / pro intervention. The best ones save the family

Giving more chances doesn't work. If they knew how to end their addictive behavior they would have done it already. Admitting one needs help and getting help doesn't mean one has to admit they are also powerless

Drug and alcohol addiction is characterized by obsessive and compulsive behavior, temporarily out of the immediate control of the individual. Cravings and triggers can drive a person to abuse again. Do they have new skills, improved ability and greater strength to overcome these cravings and triggers? How will they gain them? Ending addiction requires new abilities, skills and ending their cravings, depression and guilt without covering those up.

FIGHTING ADDICTIONS - HOW TO HELP A PERSON OVERCOME ADDICTIONS

Addition to drugs, alcohol and other substance abuse takes place generally at the time your child joins college. For the college student, it is the first time when you are free of all restraint, and generally, you are part of a group of people who are experiencing freedom from all angles, since you have a limited college class time, and the rest of the time is yours.

Yes, in school too, in recent times, drugs, alcohol and other substance abuse has been reported.

There are two ways of handling such children and teenagers. One is to try and talk to them about the various effects it has on their life and how it affects their brains, and the ruin it leads to as a person. But such an effort by a parent generally is most of the time unheard, and the addition continues.

There are other methods like getting your child into a de-addition program. There are a number of institutions that specialize in providing treatment for addition to drugs, alcohol and substance abuse. But these are not enough.

First and foremost, it is the user, your child, who has to make up the mind to give it up. There may be a variety of reasons as to why they have become addicted. It can be to be part of a peer group, or simply because they may be frustrated with some part of their life. And to get to that part of their life which triggers such addictive behavior is quite difficult. It can range from a comment made by someone whom they considered close, a family which has broken up, siblings who have broken up with the addict, and so many causes.

In all these kinds of cases of additions, there are two parties who have to work together to wean them from this social and medical evil. Most people tend to treat these habit forming addiction as a social disorder. In fact, it is a disease much like the flu, virus, colds and cough. Instead of physical symptoms, the symptoms relate to psychology. Most people who suffer from such abuse come from broken homes, frustration faced by them in school, college or in social standing.

Most of the time they require lots of love and care. Once addicted, it is very difficult to break the vicious cycle. Any wrong use of words or even silence can drive them again back into the arms of that addiction. A great deal of tender loving care is required, and a whole host of supportive measures are required. Friends, neighbors, relatives need to rally around and help the addict. There are various community groups which help families to cope with this kind of addiction, and generally there is a sociologist and psychologist who try and help.

But the real effort has to be made by the addict themselves. They need to understand that getting into addiction is a one way street, the end of which is the end of life itself. While the end of life is not in their hands, they would have ruined themselves. Not having enough money to buy more and more of that addictive substance, they would tend to lie, steal, or even sell their bodies to get that addictive substance.

They are emotionally demoralized. They need love and affection. They need care. They need counseling. Teenagers generally rebel against any advice given. They need to realise themselves that the addiction is something that CAN be cured. All it requires is the will power to resist the urge. The urge becomes so strong that the patient, which the addicts are, can do anything to get the dope they want.

To get their self-respect back, their will to be brought back, sometimes they need to spend time in special institutions which try to break their habits by certain restraints, apart from medication. This requires specially skilled people who are either addicts themselves earlier, and have now reformed.

For persons who still have not reached that stage, it is important for them to realize that the choice lies with them, and that while others can help, it is more important that they themselves make the choice to come back to the normal world, and to face it boldly.

In helping these people, their parents, siblings, neighbors and others need to exercise tremendous amounts of patience, understanding, and be careful in their words for the withdrawal symptoms of an addict is such that anything slightly out of place WILL be misunderstood and back they go.. so it's a balance that has to be struck. Most times, getting medical care in a facility is the best chance to get back into a normal life.

Is Someone Close to You an Alcoholic?

Alcohol is by far the most-abused substance in the United States. Its role as an abused substance is made all the more prevalent still due to the fact that it is one of the few legal, recreational drugs. According to the Center for Disease Control and Prevention, over 60% of adults in the U.S drank alcohol this past year. Over one-third of those people regularly consume five or more drinks in one sitting.

In my work as a counselor, I unfortunately come across alcoholism fairly regularly. It's hard for those of us who occasionally take a benign, social drink to perceive just how bad alcoholism can be. Sadly, I see alcohol's damaging affects far too regularly. The devastating impact it can have on the body, family and general lives of those afflicted is enough to make me stop and think every time a waiter offers me glass of wine or a buddy hands me a cold one on a hot summer day. Alcoholism occurs regularly and often right under our noses. Denial of the illness is one of its most characteristic symptoms. It is for that reason that the Alcoholics Anonymous program's first step is such: "We admitted we were powerless over alcohol-that our lives had become unmanageable."

If you suspect, even slightly, that a friend or loved one has a problem with alcoholism, seek help immediately. But how can you tell for certain? Such accusations are weighty and given the sensitive nature of the issue, you will want to be sure before potentially igniting an uncomfortable situation.

If you suspect a friend, relative or loved one has succumbed to alcoholism, but are uncertain, here are a few signs to help inform your decision to seek counsel or assistance. Remember alcoholism can be dangerous, even fatal, so you should not hesitate to seek help for your friend immediately.

* Health Symptoms are Noticeable - Certain ailments are often prevalent in alcoholics, even in the short term. Symptoms of hangover are nausea, stomach and head pain that often accompany dehydration. Oftentimes

unconsciousness, blackout and amnesia can occur after a moderate dose of alcohol. Long-term affects can be far more serious and can include high blood pressure, brain damage and liver failure. So if you've seen someone close to you regularly suffering from the short-term health problems equated with alcohol, do or say something lest the problems escalate.

* Your Relationships is Affected by Their Drinking - Often drinking is the alcoholic's first priority. This can be painful, because your loved one's drinking seems to take precedence, even before your relationship. This should be a red flag to you: The drinking has gone too far.

* School and Work are Suffering Due to Drinking- Drinking is too often the most important aspect of the alcoholic's life. School or work are some of the first and more obvious things that begin to suffer as a result. If your loved one has begun to miss deadlines or school assignments and begun to slack at work or school, he may have fallen pray to alcohol abuse.

* Psychological Issues - Alcohol is often used as a means to self-medicate depression, anxiety, irritability and insomnia. Alas, drinking often aggravates and worsens these problems. An alcoholic will often attempt to cover up these self-medicating tendencies, so be wary and sensitive when approaching these issues.

* Inability to Stop - Perhaps the most obvious indicator that a true problem exists. An ordinary person can stop drinking, an alcoholic cannot. People addicted to alcohol suffer from cravings as well as withdrawal symptoms when they don't drink. If you perceive these symptoms, don't hesitate to intervene.

Of course, the most dangerous symptom remains plain old denial. This is oftentimes the greatest hurdle to overcome when confronting a friend or loved one who abuses alcohol. Alcoholics generally believe they that they still retain control over the situation. Only once a problem has been acknowledged can help and intervention become truly effective. In the counseling work I've done with alcoholics, I always do my best to gently convince the alcoholic that his or her drinking has gotten out of hand. The most effective convincing though comes from close friends and caring family members. Nothing hits home to someone afflicted with alcohol abuse or addiction as seeing the damage they've wrought upon those they love most.

If you've begun to suspect someone close to you of succumbing to alcoholism, don't wait. Seek the help of a professional counselor who can advise you on the best course of action. Be discreet and subtle, but don't let your suspicions go unchecked. Get involved. Your decision to do so could save a life.

Alcohol And The Liver

No heavy drinker can afford to underestimate the problems of damaging their liver. In some cases, those with cirrhosis may be fortunate enough to receive a liver transplant, but this is only likely to be granted if the individual concerned remains completely dry for at least six months beforehand. So anyone who has been abusing alcohol for any period of time is well advised to consult their GP, who can use scans and blood tests to assess what damage you have caused. They can also provide timely advice on how to cut down and adopt healthier drinking patterns which can reduce the chances of liver disease and other alcohol related problems such as hypertension and depression. Unfortunately, unlike with many other medical conditions, the early signs of liver disease are not always easy to spot by the drinker themselves because the liver has very few nerve ends, and by the time the drinker is feeling any significant pain it could well be too late to make a recovery. If spotted early enough, however, mild liver damage can be fairly straightforward to overcome because the liver has a remarkable ability to repair itself. So seeking professional advice at the first possibility if you know you have been drinking well in excess of the government's recommended safety guidelines is the surest way of avoiding a death sentence.

Your liver is responsible for processing the alcohol you drink and eliminating it from the body by breaking it down into water, gas and fat. But this is only one of hundreds of important jobs it does. So it starts experiencing considerable strain if you drink heavily. It essentially has to start doing overtime if you drink more than about half a pint of beer or its equivalent an hour.

Just as some employees who are continuously asked to work unreasonable hours handle the strain better than others, no two livers can be guaranteed to react to the excess demands placed on them in exactly the same way. The difference between a disgruntled employee and a disgruntled liver is that the employee is likely to make their feelings known at a relatively early stage.

If you accidentally put your finger on an oven hotplate, you are likely to take it away again pretty quickly. Unfortunately, the liver has no such built-in safety mechanism because it has very few nerve ends. It is therefore quite possible that a problem drinker will not experience any physical pain until they have entered the final stages of alcoholic liver disease, by which time it could be too late to make a recovery.

For this reason it is important that anyone who suspects they have been drinking too heavily for a prolonged period should seek medical advice. Trying to feel your liver at the bottom of your rib cage is unlikely to tell you anything, but doctors can detect damage by using blood tests and, if required, scans.

Fortunately, if liver damage can be spotted early enough it can normally be reversed, because most livers are sufficiently tough to withstand serious abuse by replacing damaged cells with healthy ones. Two or three years of heavy drinking, or 10 or 20 years of drinking slightly over the government's recommended guidelines, can cause significant damage without being accompanied by any symptoms. Although, if you then stop drinking or cut down to safe levels, the liver may be able to carry on working.

There is, however, the danger that the liver will eventually conclude that enough is enough. The final stages of liver disease occur when it finally runs out of healthy cells and develops cirrhosis. Once it has developed cirrhosis, your liver can't recover, although you can prevent further damage and increase your chances of survival if you stop drinking.

In the very final stages of cirrhosis, the liver becomes so damaged that the whole body becomes poisoned by waste products which the liver has become unable to deal with. This will lead to the failure of major organs, which is likely to prove fatal. The dying process is also likely to be very painful.

THE GREAT HOAX BETWEEN ALCOHOL AND YOUR HEALTH

It's not that you have been lied to. You've just been told a limited portion of the facts. The behemoth multinational corporations that market alcoholic beverages watch their stock prices soar every time a study is published demonstrating that alcohol is good for your health. And drinkers, many of whom are in denial that they have a problem or are in the early stage of alcoholism, can rationalize that their addiction is actually good for them. Is it really? Mark Twain is quoted as saying that there are three kinds of falsehood: lies, damn lies, and statistics. So it is with data presented by the popular media regarding alcohol:

• The alcohol corporations' spin doctors tell you only what they want you to know.

• They have narrow and unrealistic definitions of terms that don't match the public perceptions of drinking.

Narrowly defined, "moderate alcohol consumption" lowers health risk from cardiovascular disease. But it raises risk for various cancers, hepatitis, osteoporosis, immune suppression, accidents, and suicide. They don't tell you that part. With selective filtration of the facts, the liquor industry continues to advocate alcohol as a beneficial part of a healthful diet. Moderate and heavy drinkers, with denial and rationalization fully operational, proclaim alcohol to be the fountain of youth.

In stark contrast, the health hazards that tobacco use causes outrages the American public. Class action suits, public service announcements, prohibition of smoking in public places, and health warnings on packages attest to the increased public awareness and sentiment against tobacco use. Like alcohol lobbyists today, tobacco lobbyists at one time hid the devastating health risks from the public.

Alcohol is contributory to nine different types of cancer and gastro esophageal reflux disease (GERD). Its role in producing fetal alcohol syndrome (FAS) accounts for 11 percent of the money spent for the treatment of mental retardation in this country. It is a leading cause of osteoporosis, suppresses the immune system, and is a major factor in highway deaths, spousal and child abuse, and homicide. Smokers harm only themselves and their immediate family through secondhand exposure. Alcohol harms randomly on the streets and highways of America and, in an ever-widening circle, the family and friends of the alcoholic. So why doesn't the package labeling on alcoholic beverages really reflect the extent of these hazards? It does... somewhat:

Government Warning: (1) According to the surgeon general, women should not drink alcoholic beverages during pregnancy because of the risk of birth defects. (2) Consumption of alcoholic beverages impairs your ability to drive a car or operate machinery and may cause health problems.

HOW ALCOHOLIC BEHAVIOR DESTROYS YOUR TRUST

The recurring theme is a pattern of alcoholic behavior which includes being irresponsible and lying. Here is a recent case from my practice that illustrates the difficulties of having a boyfriend with an alcohol problem.

T.R. is 24 years old and has been dating a recovering alcoholic for six months. They get along well and she has been very pleased that he treats her 4 year-old son in a loving and kind way. Her son has become very fond of him. Several weeks ago, T.R. was at a family dinner with her alcoholic boyfriend, her parents, and some close friends. Her boyfriend excused himself from the table. He never returned! She called him multiple times on his cell phone, but he did not respond. She did not know what to think. She felt a range of emotions including anger, resentment, worry, embarrassment (how do you explain this to your family) and panic.

She did not hear from him for 2 days! When he finally contacted her, he told her some crazy excuse why he had left the dinner without telling anyone. She knew he was lying. She confronted him about having an alcohol relapse. He denied it and became very defensive.

This case is a variation of the following themes I hear: he disappeared, he lost his cell phone, his car broke down etc. The other common scenarios are the girlfriend finds empty alcohol bottles hidden in drawers, her boyfriend comes in smashed at 3AM, he promises to quit drinking alcohol, but continues to drink.

Typical alcoholic behavior impacts the victim (you) in negative ways. Alcoholic behavior includes lying, hiding drinking, not being responsible about keeping in touch, getting defensive about an alcohol relapse when confronted, and being in denial that alcohol is the dominant force in his life (interfering with his personal life and his work).

Anyone with an active alcohol problem is focused on drinking alcohol and is not focused on a relationship. His main relationship is with a bottle of alcohol. A person who is actively drinking alcohol or using drugs is unable to meet the needs of his partner in a consistent way. He believes he needs alcohol (his brain is alcohol dependent) and you think you need him.

The more alcoholic behavior you are willing to put up with, the more you are demonstrating that you are addicted to him, in your own way.If you want a stable, healthy, and happy relationship, find someone else. If he decides to go into alcoholic recovery, it usually takes a year of sobriety to be able to handle a romantic relationship.

Marriages to an alcoholic husband tend to be very stormy and difficult. If you go on to marry your alcoholic boyfriend, you most likely have issues with your own self-esteem that should be addressed. Try attending Al-Anon meetings to get some perspective about your unhealthy relationship and learn how to set appropriate boundaries.

HOW TO RECOVER FROM ADDICTION

Alcoholism, Drug Abuse- Challenges Facing Family, Friends and the Addict in Britain

What are some of the challenges facing Britains who are tackling problems of alcohol abuse and drug addiction in their lives. In the UK, the difficulties facing addicts, alcoholics and their families are similar to others all over the world, but each culture has its own set of unique challenges. Learn to spot these in your home environment and get closer to the truth of the problem and how to recover from it. We look at things everyday but do we actually see how they are influencing our lives.

How Do You Recover From Drug Addiction and Alcoholism?

Deciding something must be done about the problem

Not waiting for the fabled "Rock Bottom"

Finding your courage to not give up

Giving the addict or alcoholic hope to get better

Educating yourself on drug addicted behaviour and alcoholism

Educating yourself on drug and alcohol rehab program alternatives and success rates

Intervention, what to do, who can help

Spotting social pressures, family and friends-Truth vs Marketing Lies

Alcohol and Marketing- The Truth vs. The Lie

It seems that alcohol is everywhere. In my local upscale fitness club in Central London, I am bombarded with wine adverts from the moment I walk in. At my local foodstore, it is 25% off wine bottles if I buy the alcohol in bulk. The pubs are always busy and almost always open. The coffee houses close early. Anytime is the right time for a drink, or so it seems. For those trying to enjoy a drug free and alcohol free life, this is a huge challenge in the fight to stay clean and sober.

Recently, one of the trendy London based radio stations just renamed themselves after a very well known brand of Vodka. Funny thing, when I think of that radio station, I also think of alcohol. Coincidence? Maybe...

Marketing Tells Us Alcohol Will Improve Your Life- See How?

Many primetime TV shows are sponsored by alcohol companies. Many programs make sure they show drinking alcohol and sex; drinking and having fun; drinking alcohol and sports. Drinking alcohol is promoted as going hand in hand with anything worthwhile in life. The alcohol producers seem to be winning as many consumers, are buying into that marketing strategy.

Honestly has alcohol bettered your life? Does it make you happier, stronger, more confident, healthy? Alcohol does not equal happiness and prosperity. It is a lie. We know this by all the pain and destroyed lives, that surround us. We know this by the 1.2 million violent crimes committed annually in England associated with alcohol.

Binging is socially accepted as a norm. If you live in the UK, I'm sure that this is familiar and so much so that most think nothing of it. Britain has a reputation as being a nation of binge drinkers. A sad truth that many would hope to dispel.

In the Borough of Camden London alone, there are an estimated 45,000 "hazardous drinkers" and then there are the estimated 11,000 "harmful and dependent drinkers". I think that the biggest challenge facing alcoholics is the Social Pressures to Drink Alcohol and Use Drugs. Take a moment to notice the way in which we get bombarded with alcohol publicity and that is one step closer to beating the problem.

What Is The Truth About Help And Recovery?

Honest help does make a relationship better, sex better, health better, work better. Being told that these things can be achieved in life through alcohol and drug use is not an honest effort to help but to harm. Look around your environment and see these social pressures for what they are. With that clarity, find the strength to follow the other steps to recovery and a drug and alcohol free life

TRAIT OF AN ALCOHOLIC/ADDICT

What does it mean to be an alcoholic? How do you know when problem drinking has become an addiction? These are some of the most difficult and challenging questions a problem drinker faces, and before he accepts that he is indeed an alcoholic, the drinker is beyond help.

Here, is a check list of criteria that defines most alcoholics. Firstly an alcoholic is completely powerless over alcohol and has no defence against the first drink. Do you find that on the days when you try as hard as you can to not drink, that you wind up drunk anyway?

How many times on your way home have you wandered into a bar, off licence or other place that sells booze, sure that 'this time it'll be different' and if you have had a problem in the past 'it's OK now'?

Alcoholics all have an internal civil war raging 24/7, they struggle with their desire to drink and a guilty knowledge of the consequences of drinking. Alcoholics find themselves exhausted by this ongoing battle, they find themselves constantly living in shame over their 'weakness' and constantly hoping that they won't be found out by others.

This means that alcoholics need to constantly lie, lie to themselves, their loved ones, their friends, employers and acquaintances. The difference between the reality of their situation and the story that they spin to themselves and others results in a great pain that they must carry around with them.

The fantasy world the addicted drinker has to create in order to sustain a lifestyle that is slowly destroying them as akin to a certain type of madness.

No one can tell an alcoholic that they are one, they must decide for themselves. I have known drinkers to debate the semantics of their condition up to their institutionalisation and premature death, because it is an illness with a life of its own, leaving the decision about whether one is or is not an alcoholic down to the drinker can often be fatal.

Many alcoholics will do anything to prevent themselves from admitting their true nature because they know that when they do, the game is up, there can be no more self-deception.

When an addict admits the truth and accepts defeat there can be no more lies and the addiction is dealt a serious blow, a light of truth is shone upon it and it can never quite have the same hold over the addict again.

If you know that you are powerless over alcohol, but if you still have a mental obsession with drinking, if you are thinking about alcohol now, if you feel that you can't cope without a drink to help you through the day, you may well be an alcoholic, but it is your decision to make.

ALCOHOLISM SCREENING TESTS AND THE CAGE TEST

The use of alcohol is acceptable in most societies. Even as children we see advertisements that make alcohol look fun and sexy, so we accept it as a part of life, and when we are old enough we are left to self-administer this drug, how, when and where we like. Most people enjoy an occasional drink, a few drinks at a party, after work, or a glass of wine with a meal and have no problems. Others, for many complex reasons, find that they start to drink heavily, or more frequently. Still other worry if they could perhaps be starting down a slope into addiction.

Alcoholism screening tests have been devised for those of us who are not sure if we are alcohol-dependent or not. The CAGE questionnaire is a simple, four question test that we can use to gauge if our alcohol use is not simply use, but abuse, and of course being honest is the key to finding the right answer.

The first question in the CAGE test asks if you feel that you should reduce your alcohol intake. This will involve a certain amount of introspection, you will have to think about situations you may have gotten into after consuming too much alcohol, such as being drunk and waking up on the floor, for example.

If someone who is close to you has said something about your drinking and you have reacted either defensively or angrily, the second question addresses that scenario. If you did react in a way that is out of character for you, then you may be in denial. It can be hard too face the fact that you may be drinking too heavily, or at inappropriate times.

Do you feel guilty? Have you been late home from work and lied that you were working late, when in fact you were in a bar? Did you have several beers, but lied and said you only had a couple of drinks? You lied as a defense - you have an addiction, and you are not willing to admit to it. Again you are in denial and that guilt comes along with denial.

The last question asks if you wake up in the morning wanting a drink, to either steady your nerves or help to get rid of a hangover - the hair of the dog as it's called. The CAGE test is a very short, sharp, shock if you answer yes to all the questions - you need to seek help. There are many other, and much longer alcoholism screening tests, but there is one online developed by Johns Hopkins University Hospital, that contains only three questions. Answering yes to all three questions is a sure sign that you are becoming, or have become, alcohol-dependent.

Taking any of these tests voluntarily and honestly is a good sign that you are worried about your own physical health and well-being. Congratulations. The major part of the battle with alcohol is realizing that you have a problem - chances are with the right help, a change of habits and a positive attitude, you can be on the road to recovery quickly.

The use of alcohol is acceptable in most societies. Even as children we see advertisements that make alcohol look fun and sexy, so we accept it as a part of life, and when we are old enough we are left to self-administer this drug, how, when and where we like. Most people enjoy an occasional drink, a few drinks at a party, after work, or a glass of wine with a meal and have no problems. Others, for many complex reasons, find that they start to drink heavily, or more frequently. Still other worry if they could perhaps be starting down a slope into addiction.

Alcoholism screening tests have been devised for those of us who are not sure if we are alcohol-dependent or not. The CAGE questionnaire is a simple, four question test that we can use to gauge if our alcohol use is not simply use, but abuse, and of course being honest is the key to finding the right answer.

The first question in the CAGE test asks if you feel that you should reduce your alcohol intake. This will involve a certain amount of introspection, you will have to think about situations you may have gotten into after consuming too much alcohol, such as being drunk and waking up on the floor, for example.

If someone who is close to you has said something about your drinking and you have

261

reacted either defensively or angrily, the second question addresses that scenario. If you did react in a way that is out of character for you, then you may be in denial. It can be hard too face the fact that you may be drinking too heavily, or at inappropriate times.

Do you feel guilty? Have you been late home from work and lied that you were working late, when in fact you were in a bar? Did you have several beers, but lied and said you only had a couple of drinks? You lied as a defense - you have an addiction, and you are not willing to admit to it. Again you are in denial and that guilt comes along with denial.

The last question asks if you wake up in the morning wanting a drink, to either steady your nerves or help to get rid of a hangover - the hair of the dog as it's called. The CAGE test is a very short, sharp, shock if you answer yes to all the questions - you need to seek help. There are many other, and much longer alcoholism screening tests, but there is one online developed by Johns Hopkins University Hospital, that contains only three questions. Answering yes to all three questions is a sure sign that you are becoming, or have become, alcohol-dependent.

Taking any of these tests voluntarily and honestly is a good sign that you are worried about your own physical health and well-being. Congratulations. The major part of the battle with alcohol is realizing that you have a problem - chances are with the right help, a change of habits and a positive attitude, you can be on the road to recovery quickly.

COMMON LIES PEOPLE USE TO MINIMIZE ALCOHOLISM OR ADDICTION

Addiction takes a powerful hold not only on the addicted person, but on their loved ones and family members. Both the addicted person and their significant others often fight the label of addiction because of the old and highly inaccurate belief that addiction is simply a matter of weak will or moral failing.

In order for someone to get help, they have to first recognize there is a problem. Sometimes it is the pressure from friends and family that finally moves someone to get the help they need. Here are 10 common lies we tell ourselves to minimize an addiction, either our own addiction or that of a family member, which can delay getting treatment.

1. I can quit anytime I want

This is the common claim of alcoholics and addicts. It's hard to disprove it because if you say, "Then quit," they will say they don't feel like it right now, but they could if they wanted to.

2. He is under a lot of stress, so that's the only reason he's drinking so much

This is one of the most common excuses for excessive drinking or drug use. It is often accompanied by statements such as, "If I had a better job," "If my wife didn't nag me," "If I wasn't so financially stressed," and similar explanations as to why someone "needs" to drink or use drugs.

3. My drug use or drinking is my business; it doesn't hurt anyone else

Nothing could be further from the truth. The addict is moody, unpredictable, unreliable, and sometimes an embarrassment. They sometimes drive while intoxicated, making it everyone's business. They put a burden on the health-care system due to the impact addiction has on their body and brain. They can't possibly be as productive or work or as good a parent as they could without drugs and alcohol affecting their abilities. Drug addiction and alcoholism take an enormous financial toll on society, and a big emotional toll on families.

4. She only drinks on the weekends

Binge drinking is a common form of alcoholism. Unfortunately, it tends to be accompanied by even more denial than you find with daily drinkers. You may have heard the story of the mother who killed herself, some of her children and sibling's children, as well as another driver and his passenger while driving back from a camping trip intoxicated on alcohol and marijuana. All her family members expressed shock, saying she didn't really drink that much.

There has been a growing trend of young mothers drinking in a way that disguises the problem. They might drink alone during the day, or binge drink to let lose on the weekends. A person does not have to drink every day to have a problem with alcohol that requires treatment.

5. That DUI was unfair - I wasn't that drunk

DUIs are serious business. When you drive a car under the influence of alcohol or drugs you are not at 100%, regardless of how low the blood alcohol content (BAC) is. You are driving a lethal ton or so of metal. You need to be totally in control. Occasionally a normal drinker makes a mistake and drives after they've had one drink, but they did it on an empty stomach, have a low body weight, or just didn't wait long enough. However, if the BAC is well over the legal limit or if they get a second DUI, it's no longer just a single case of poor judgment. Normal drinkers get the message after one DUI. The embarrassment and financial cost are enough to deter future incidents. The alcoholic does not have the ability to make good decisions once they drink, and will tend to get more DUIs.

6. The doctor prescribed all those different medications, so they must be fine

Not all doctors prescribe with care, and not all patients are honest with their doctors. Opiates are the most commonly abused prescription drug, along with anti-anxiety and sleeping pills. If you are taking multiple pills that have the effect of suppressing the central nervous system, you are treading dangerous waters. It's important to look at how many prescriptions the person takes that are classified as a Schedule II, III, or IV controlled substance; taking many different mood-altering drugs is typically very risky and unhealthy behavior. If the person has multiple doctors writing these prescriptions, or goes to different pharmacies to fill them, these should set off warning bells.

7. I don't drink in the morning, so I can't be an alcoholic

This is one of those old myths, similar to the I-only-drink-on-weekends myth. When you drink or what time you start really is secondary to how much you drink, how much it affects your behavior and life, and how hard it is to stay abstinent from alcohol.

8. He isn't that bad; I know people who drink a lot more than that

Comparing how one person drinks to another is a real trap for some people. Everyone has a different metabolism and various factors that influence how they are affected by alcohol. More important, how other people abuse alcohol isn't really your concern. Your concern should be how alcohol impacts your life. You might say this excuse is akin to saying you've only had two heart attacks and you know a guy who's had four, so you really don't have heart disease.

9. She has a great job and never calls in sick, so she can't have a problem

High-functioning alcoholics can get away with abusing substances a lot longer than other people. There are people who just seem able to push through their addiction and maintain an outward appearance of being just fine. Having a good job, lots of money, or great kids does not mean you don't have an alcohol problem. Examine the areas of your life that could be better if you weren't under the influence. That's a more accurate way to assess the situation.

10. I only drink beer and wine, not the hard stuff

Old myths die hard, and this is one of those stories alcoholics tell themselves so they can keep on drinking. If you drink six beers every night, you may as well knock back six shots of whisky. They are equivalent. What you drink is not important, it's how you drink and the impact it has on you, your life, and your family.

ALCOHOL AND ALCOHOLISM

Blackouts

Do not remove his bottles from their hiding place, because when he goes to hide more, it will indicate to him the extent of his drinking, if his head is sufficiently clear to identify such sickness.

Alcoholics suffer from blackouts and do not always remember where they have hidden their bottles, often concealed when drunk and he cannot remember where. Always there is the need to have yet another hidey-hole and we forget. Sometimes it is even better to bring one out of deep hiding, because you will most probably know where most of them are anyway, and put something for him into one of his more obvious and easily accessible hiding places, before he wrecks the house looking for it. He will, you know!

Blackouts need an explanation. In a blackout does not mean that they are lying down unconscious on the floor. Alcoholics can be walking about or sitting quietly, apparently having a reasonably normal conversation with you, whatever a normal conversation is with a drunk, drinking, and then later, when they are not drinking, remember nothing about it.

This is a blackout.

They can promise in all sincerity so that you will believe them to take you all to the beach in the morning and then in the morning, when you are all kitted up, ready to go, he arrives downstairs looking like something out of a horror movie and nobody is going anywhere. He knows nothing at all about it.

And, you are not going anywhere. For sure.

Also, it is often during these blackouts that the most violent scenes take place, and you wonder desperately why they do not believe you when you confront them with what they have said or done the next day, or in the morning, and you start to wonder if you are going out of your mind.

One handy thing to remember is not to put alcoholics to bed when they are in a state of collapse, as they think that all is well when they awaken to orderly surroundings, and once again when you try to tell them what they did, and what happened, they do not believe you, as they were most likely in a blackout again.

Waking up in bed, with clothes neatly and tidily folded on the chair, gives the impression that everything is alright, and this can often be far from the truth.

If they fall asleep on the stairs, or on the settee, or on the floor, or slumped over the table just make sure that their clothing, their tie, belt, collar and any other tight items are undone, and that they are in a safe position and not lying directly on their backs, so that they hopefully will not choke on their own vomit.

Although you may be displeased with him, do this carefully and with love, for under all that alcohol and unacceptable behaviour he is still your partner, the one you married, and love and perhaps sleep with, and then when he awakes at three or four or five or six in the morning, perhaps on the kitchen floor, hopefully not still in a blackout, he may once again be able to see the extent of his drinking, and where it has taken him.

He cannot help his drinking.

He is powerless over his drinking.

He has no control over his intake of alcohol.

He might make the decision right then to do something about it.

No-one can ever know when that moment will arrive.

That moment of "Had enough of it all ....."

Remember that the basic plan behind all of our suggestions is to make him aware, and not to criticise or judge him. We know that he is sick, but he does not, and we can all help when he is ready.

By making him responsible for all of the things that he does when he is drinking we are doing the very best that we can for him. If we keep making him responsible for his conduct he will hopefully say one day "Enough" and put down the glass.

Everyone has a chance at this from time to time, but we do not make things tough enough for them, and they keep on having people doing things for them, and picking up the pieces all the time, so they do not have to stop drinking. As long as you continue to pick up the pieces, that is doing things for him, putting him to bed, giving him money, lying for him, fetching his booze from the off licence, cashing his cheques for him, going to the cash machine for him, jumping for him, dancing for him, and so on - nothing is more certain than that he will continue to drink.

Stop it.

Try one or two things .....

Do not continue to try to conceal what is happening in your lives, in your family and in your home. This is like trying to stop the rain coming down. Be honest. Stop denying what is happening.

Make him totally responsible for his drinking.

Make him totally responsible for the results of his drinking, no matter what they may be. Perhaps falling over in the street. Drinking and driving. Court appearances. Bailiffs coming.

Do not cover up anything for him. Stop lying for him. Do not apologise for him.

Try not to argue with him or to bring up controversial subjects for discussion with him when he is drinking. You cannot win an argument with a drunk. We know how difficult these things are but try them when you judge it right. You only will be the judge. No-one knows him and his moods better. You will know, better than anyone, when it is safe to talk to him about certain things.

When he is drinking or drunk and drinking and he wants to bring some controversial subject up for discussion, try saying "We will discuss this tomorrow morning" - or - "We will have a talk when you are not drinking!" Be positive. Agree. Tomorrow. He will be pleased with that. You agreeing.

Try not to use the expression "When you are sober" for it is not recommended. This implies that he is drunk, and even if he is, it is judgmental and he will deny it, and so an argument ensues.

Using "Not whilst you are drinking" most especially if he has glass-in-hand, refers to an established fact, and is not an opinion.

Try "Not whilst you are drinking" then, it can sometimes just stop things right there.

You cannot, in any case, successfully argue with a drunk who is drinking.

You will already be aware that your opinions are always questionable. Worthless.

You will already also be aware that your answers and comments are always wrong.

Not sometimes, as with reasonable people, but always wrong.

He has no thought processing that will allow you to be right.

While the drinking is going on all that we are trying to do is cool it. Cool things down, so that you do not find yourself snapping back and buying the full package.

LYING, DRINKING AND BEING LEFT BEHIND

The United States is one of the few countries that have recognized that many of its citizens have trouble with regulating alcohol intake. This may be in part because other countries train their children to drink alcohol responsibly earlier than the 21 year waiting period found in the United States. There are many signs of alcohol abuse that play into getting a person help.

One sign of alcohol abuse is if a person is out on the town and they cannot just stick to one drink. When driving, monitoring a healthy inflow of alcohol is paramount to controlling someone's abilities. By not being able to control intake and always saying, "Yea, it's ok, just one more," a person can tell that they have started down the path towards alcoholism.

Another way to tell if someone is developing an alcohol problem is by them feeling guilty or ashamed about drinking. When someone feels ashamed, they have a guilty conscience and can now see that they have lost control over themselves and need the drink. When someone loses control over how much they imbibe, they are well down the path towards an unhealthy addiction to alcohol.

If a person has ever blacked out or passed out as a result of drinking, or constantly needs a drink to beat a hangover, they have a problem. Blacking out occurs when the human body ingests more alcohol than the filtration system of the body can handle. Regurgitating during a black out session has led to many deaths and is quite dangerous. Blacking out is a serious occurrence that must be curbed immediately.

When a person lies about drinking, but loved ones know the truth, it is a sign that there could be a problem. Lying about drinking plays back into feeling ashamed and means someone is trying to cover up their tracks. When family and friends pose an intervention or are constantly telling someone to get help, they should listen. Intervention is a great way to get addicts to realize that they have a problem.

While alcoholism is no laughing matter, our society almost welcomes addictive behavior. Symptoms of alcohol abuse include not being able to just have one, lying about it, interventions, blacking out, or feeling guilty or ashamed of drinking. Seek help for anyone who exhibits these characteristics because they definitely need help. However, the first step in making them understand that they need to acknowledge that they do indeed have a problem.

HOW TO HANDLE
ADOLESCENT LYING

Sad to say, everyone lies sometimes. We lie by not telling someone about something that we know would make them unhappy (e.g. "Your mother said she's always liked your sister best!"). We lie to avoid hurting people's feelings about their choice of clothes, hair color, or companions. But, generally, most of us want very much to live lives of honesty, particularly with those who are closest to us. However, with adolescents, lies can escalate and become the first line of defense against parental control. Typically, these lies take the form of 3 W's - Where, Who, and What.

The Where is often the most difficult to pin down. Because of cell phone use, teens today can respond to a parent phone call from anywhere on the planet! So parents who keep tabs on their teen by having them call in or by calling them on their cell phone can be easily mislead. A classic ploy is for a youngster to tell his parents that he is going to a friend's house for a sleep over and then leaves that house to attend a party. The ease with which this happens is amazing. All the young co-conspirators require is permission to go out from the host parent (if that parent is even at home). They do not need to say they will be attending a party but, instead, going to a movie or another friend's home.

The second W, the Who, is often misrepresented when the adolescent knows that his parents do not approve of certain friends. For some teens, the fact that parents dislike their companions is actually reinforcing! It adds a sense of adventure and rebellion at a time when hormones and mental development are affecting judgment and self-control. So the savvy teen plans his outings carefully by arranging to be seen or heard talking about activities with an acceptable friend and then meeting up with the unacceptable friend at another location. For this operation to succeed, the entire group has to work cooperatively, covering for each other if parents call or ask questions at a later time.

Then the What becomes an issue. Spending time at a party or associating with questionable characters is not in and of itself a problem. The real problem occurs when teens use their stolen moments to engage in activities that endanger themselves or others. For example, it is a rare party that does not have alcohol and drugs available. That is not to say that all teens will partake, but when mood altering substances are available, bad things can happen. Physical accidents, unwanted sexual intimacies, driving under the influence, and drug or alcohol overdoses happen frequently when adolescents are allowed to use alcohol and drugs. Sometimes, it is the parent hosts who look the other way or who provide the alcohol - excusing this behavior by the false rational that it allows them to monitor what their adolescent is doing in the safety of the home environment.

So how does a concerned parent monitor their teen without resorting to becoming an obsessive parent? Monitoring is an ongoing, multifaceted process. First, and most important, parents must be aware of what their teen is doing. Even the most trustworthy, competent adolescent can slip when parents are never home. Parents need to touch base with teens on a daily basis. That means making time to talk with them even when they resist family activities. The need for 'alone time' is very common with teens, but every teen should be required to participate in some form of family time.

Second, parents need to be very clear about family expectations with respect to underage drinking, sexual activities, and drug use. Forbidding attendance at group functions and parties can lead to subversive behavior. A more practical solution is to ensure that the adolescent has an emergency plan for leaving or for contacting parents if the situation is not comfortable. It is also important that parents contact the host prior to the event and determine whether parents (not an older sibling or cousin) will be present and share the same values regarding illegal substances use. This last factor is a must despite the fact that your teen may object. In fact, the wise parent has a parent network to rely upon for information and feedback regarding teen activities in the community.

With respect to sleeping over at a friend's house, make sure the other parent will be home and will comply with your expectations regarding your teen's whereabouts. And make it very clear to your teen that trust is something that must be validated by honest actions. Trust that has been lost must be re-established by future behaviors. The logical consequence for abusing trust at a sleep over is to forbid any future visits to other's homes until such a time as responsible behaviors are demonstrated. In cases where teens have really abused parental trust by drinking or using drugs the message is that trust is a privilege and not a right. In which case, the teen becomes subject to periodic parent surprise visits to ensure that the youngster is where he says he is.

Most teens are generally responsible and honest individuals. But, keep in mind, that adolescence is a time of experimentation with new identities and behaviors. Even very well-adjusted teens can make mistakes. The key for parents is to maintain open communication, convey family values and expectations, and monitor your teen's whereabouts. In the end, most adolescents grow up to be responsible, taxpaying, lawn mowing, decent citizens who lead responsible lives.

TREATMENT FOR ALCOHOL POISONING

Alcohol poisoning needs immediate medical attention to make sure that the vital system of the body remains balanced and not impaired dangerously. Some think that the treatment is as easy as sleeping the alcohol off, but the treatment for alcohol poisoning is a bigger deal than that.

Vomiting is the easiest treatment for alcohol poisoning. When intoxication happens, the risk of choking on your own vomit is very high especially when the person is unconscious. So it is advisable to turn an unconscious person to lie sideways because this is the surest and safest position to avoid choking and ensure open airways. There are many cases of intoxication leading to death for this very reason, they are left unattended and choked during vomiting and an airway becomes clogged.

Hypothermia is when alcohol lowers the temperature of the body due to constriction of the blood vessels. Excessive levels of alcohol intake can induce this dangerous condition. Usually drunks are covered in sweat or vomit and are left lying down wet. This is a dangerous state of the body and someone can die if warned up too quickly. In emergency rooms, the treatment to alcohol poisoning is to apply warm blankets and intravenous. Giving of intravenous fluid as the treatment for alcohol poisoning can also help to rehydrate the body of possible fluid loss due to excessive sweating and vomiting. The fluid of choice is usually glucose; not only for warming and to rehydrate the body, but also to bring up the glucose level to a safe and acceptable level.

Reduced Consciousness and Confusion: Alcohol content is usually the reason for a lower oxygen level thus resulting to a weird bizarre behaviour and confusion for other people. Air management and maximizing air to reduce consciousness are the quickest treatment of alcohol poisoning. Visual observations as well as medical intervention are needed to ensure the safety of the person.

This experience makes you feel sick and their integrity and dignity can also be affected. Some people do not remember what happened when they were intoxicated and often shame themselves after the fact. Drinking should be fun and enjoyable, but excessive drinking takes the fun out of a happy occasion and risks you and your health to a permanent danger. Always remember the treatment to alcohol poisoning to know what to do the next time you encounter someone with the same problem.

People should always put in mind the quickest treatment for alcohol poisoning; know their alcohol limit and stop when they are still ahead. A wild night of confusion and drunkenness is not worth the shame and hangover you'll feel the next day.

SYMPTOMS OF ADDICTION ASSOCIATED WITH DRUG AND ALCOHOL USE

When identifying the signs of addiction, it is important to know that while drug and alcohol use and abuse each manifest themselves as different behavioral changes and inconsistencies, they share a number of commonalities. This is not meant to be an all-inclusive list of signs of drug and/or alcohol addiction, but is instead a list of the most common signs that someone is suffering from addiction.

Often, addicts and alcoholics are the last to know that they have a problem, because they cannot see the outward signs of addiction. They attempt to hide their use from loved ones, escaping to a "safe" space such as a bar after work, or a spot in the garage where they can be alone to drink or use. The addict believes that he or she is keeping the drug or alcohol use secret from everyone else, when in fact, the physical and behavioral signs of addiction are often immediately apparent.

Isolation

As noted, one of the behavioral changes associated with addiction is isolation. Addicts often cite drug or alcohol use as a way to deal with stress, or just "relax after a hard day", and will either emotionally withdraw but still partake in their substance abuse in the presence of family and friends, or solitarily by escaping to a quiet spot in the home to drink or use alone. Other signs of addiction are when addicts attempt to hide their use completely, and make lengthy trips outside of the home; for example, a five-minute trip to get a pack of cigarettes or milk from the grocery store will turn into a five hour disappearance, during which time the addicted person will have gone to a friend's house or a bar to engage in drug or alcohol use.

Akin to isolation, when a person is addicted, he or she often loses interests in hobbies and activities in which he or she used to participate. Someone who was previously interested in sports and socializing with friends in a social club or association might slowly or suddenly drop out entirely. Signs of addiction can include noticing that an addicted person stops exercising, limits seeing friends or family members, or reduces his or her participation in previously enjoyable activities - because he or she is spending so much time on drug or alcohol use.

Mood Swings

When an addicted person undergoes such a drastic change in lifestyle, mood swings are often associated signs of addiction. If drug or alcohol use has gotten to the point where someone is using all of the time, the symptoms of withdrawal can include depression, irritability, fatigue, sweating, and anxiety. When that person is using, signs of addiction can be drastic improvements in mood, or suddenly shifting from being cranky to becoming happy and upbeat. These wild mood swings are the result of the drastic changes that drug and alcohol use can have upon the body and mind, and are a highly noticeable sign of addiction.

Money Troubles

One sign of addiction that is more closely aligned with drug addiction (but can be found sometimes with alcohol addiction) is that money becomes an issue. People involved with opiates or other drugs are often scrambling to find money to support their habit. Drug use, especially on a regular basis, can become a very expensive habit to maintain and addicts will often drain a bank account, steal from family members or friends, deplete a Roth IRA or drain a 401(k) in order to support their use. Signs of addiction also include noticing that a friend or family member won't have money for staples like groceries, clothing, rent, or bills, but will often find a way to continue drug or alcohol use. A partner or roommate to someone with addiction might notice that the mutual monthly contribution to finances or utilities begins to come in late, or not at all. It may even take a few months to realize a pattern in that the addicted individual is not contributing their part of the money.

Finally, signs of addiction tend to be grouped under general deceitfulness and insincerity. Isolation, withdrawal, hiding drug and alcohol use, and stealing are all behaviors that are dishonest, and lying becomes a daily habit for individuals struggling with addiction. Rarely are people truthful about their addiction. Family members often know that something is going on, but even when they confront or approach the addicted individual about their problem, the person will deny having a problem - most often because he or she is in denial about even having a problem with drug or alcohol use and abuse.

As previously stated, this is not a complete list of signs of addiction, but rather a series of common habits and behavioral changes present in both drug and alcohol users. The degrees of addiction may vary, but the common signs of isolation, lying, and behavioral / mood changes are present in almost every single person with a substance abuse problem. If you think that you or your loved one may be struggling with drug or alcohol use and addiction, consider having a discussion about how outpatient or residential addiction treatment can help you achieve sobriety and reclaim your life.

SYMPTOMS OF ALCOHOLICS AND ALCOHOLISM COUNSELING

The biggest step to getting help for alcoholics is to understand the problems and aid the alcoholic in seeing the need for a change. This is the most difficult part to beginning the steps to becoming clean and sober. This chapter will discuss the symptoms of alcoholics and alcoholism counseling.

In the beginning family and friends begin to worry about drinking episodes of someone close and become concerned about their drinking habit which appears to become more frequent. Alcohol affects some people differently than others. Sometimes the alcoholic is not even aware of his addition and believes he can stop anytime. In fact, there are millions of alcoholics who can still manage to keep their jobs until a critical event occurs.

Many alcohol counselors believe there are some clear signs before the addiction takes over. In the beginning, there is over drinking on occasion. This is how teenagers, young adults and even senior citizens start. If you have a friend or family member who is over drinking, this would be a good time to intervene with the facts. Alcoholism is addictive and consumes a life without using carefully, thought through wisdom. This type of behavior is called risky drinking.

Alcohol abuse is the next step you can see happen to your friend. Problems related to the abuse of alcohol can be seen. Bad judgment controls the thinking of an abuser and he or she might get into fights, be inappropriate with friends and dates.

Full blown alcoholism can help you distinguish other steps just leading to the addiction step. Here are the signs you will see when an alcoholic has lost control. Some the first signs are legal involvement from a drunken driving arrests to blatant lying behavior about everything.

As the years go on and alcoholism becomes a life style. You will witness devastation in the family, job loss and serious medical problems as the alcohol causes amnesia and other thinking problems at an early middle age. Finally, alcohol related illnesses and deaths rank with the higher causes of death rated today. It is a sad and unrewarding way to live life. The only one who can create the change is the alcoholic himself.

There are many avenues for counseling alcoholics. Sometimes interventions are used to assist getting the alcoholic to accept want change enough to begin treatment. Often you hear about rehabilitation clinics where the alcoholic stays for months to get sober and continue counseling so he can return to his life and stay clean. Another avenue is daytime programs that work with the alcoholics and let them return to their homes in the evening. Another way to go is to be counseled week to week by an alcohol counselor or therapist who can be successful with some folk in this setting. A free meeting with Alcoholics Anonymous is held nightly in almost every city so people who need attention to get clean and stay sober can attend as often as needed to recover

All these rehabilitation methods have merit with the symptoms of alcohol and alcoholism counseling. The most important key to success is for the addicted drinker to make the decision to change. After becoming sober, a new life style must be created with people who care about seeing him succeed. This is where family is important, Alcoholics anonymous can be very helpful and therapists also participate in coaching the recovering alcoholic to a better life. It will take a small village to combat the problems caused by alcohol use.

THE HISTORY OF ALCOHOLICS ANONYMOUS

It was a long journey from 1934 when Bill W. was diagnosed as a hopeless alcoholic by Dr. Silkworth to the founding of Alcoholics Anonymous in 1935 almost a year later. In that time, Bill W. met Dr. Bob, his lifelong friend and companion, on the journey to sobriety. They discovered early on through the lessons of others that one of the most important keys to sobriety was sharing their experiences with another. In fact, that is how Bill W. and Dr. Bob met. Bill was in Akron on business and needed to talk to another alcoholic. After much searching he connected with Dr. Bob. An immediate and strong kinship developed and these two men forged a path that, with the help of many others, has been a gift to millions seeking recovery.

Dr. Bob and Bill W. discovered the mutuality of their predicament when they met for the first time in the home of Anne S. in May of 1935. Carrying the message of Alcoholics Anonymous was to be the work of Dr. Bob, Bill W. and an army of others for years to come. Even today the message of AA passes from one alcoholic to another as they share their stories and work the 12 Steps with the support.

The First Steps

The Twelve Steps began as "six chunks of truth" (Alcoholics Anonymous Comes of Age, p. 161) in an effort to pass on the message of AA, but Bill W. had the foresight to understand that the "literature would have to be as clear and comprehensive as possible... There must not be single loophole through which the rationalizing alcoholic would wiggle out" (Alcoholics Anonymous Comes of Age, p. 161). The purpose of the steps was to ensure that every alcoholic who picked up AA literature would be able to understand the severity of the disease and the necessity for following the steps as they are written. By doing so, the alcoholic experiences the spiritual movement that is within the steps.

Step One. We admitted we were powerless over alcohol-that our lives had become unmanageable. The first of the Twelve Steps is about recognizing one's powerless in the face of alcohol. Dr. Silkworth's work on the dilemma of alcohol as both an obsession and an allergy proved to be foundational for this step. This disease which is both obsession and allergy takes over and leaves one devastated.

Step Two. Came to believe that a Power greater than ourselves could restore us to sanity. This second step is headed toward a path of surrender which happens more fully in Step 3. This is a difficult reality for alcoholics who have depended for a great deal of time on their own failed efforts to restore themselves. And yet, an important step to take because alcoholics who work the steps begin to see that relying on something or someone greater than oneself makes recovery attainable.

Step Three. Made a decision to turn our will and our lives over to the care of God as we understood Him. Letting go and letting God means that the alcoholic is able to "lose our fear of today, tomorrow or the hereafter." (Alcoholics Anonymous, p. 63) because he or she recognizes they do not have to run the show.

Step Four. Made a searching and fearless moral inventory of ourselves. This step is about looking at one's own life and laying claim to wrongs done to self and others. Without the assurance of the presence of a High Power from Step 3, this would surely be an impossible step to complete thoroughly. Writing down resentments gives them less power and allows the alcoholic the chance to begin to let them go. Trusting in an infinite Higher Power makes this step easier because the alcoholic knows that he or she is not alone on the journey.

Step Five. Admitted to God, to ourselves, and to another human being the exact nature of our wrongs. This step requires trust in a Higher Power that another will hear the story of the alcoholic with compassion and grace, sans judgment. For many this is when a cloud is lifted and a spiritual experience begins (Alcoholics Anonymous, p. 75).

Step Six. Were entirely ready to have God remove all these defects of character. This step rests between full disclosure of one's self to another and the moment when the God of one's understanding removes all those defects that once buried the alcoholic. Willingness is key because without the willingness to ask for their removal, these defects remain.

Step Seven. Humbly asked Him to remove our shortcomings. The gift of humility is one learned and accepted by the alcoholic in recovery. Faith in something greater than one's self means having the courage to let yourself be changed for the better.

Step Eight. Made a list of all persons we had harmed, and became willing to make amends to them all. Just as Steps 6 and 7 are intricately woven together, so it is true of Steps 8 and 9. This step is about preparing for the work to follow. It is important to take time to reflect on the amends to be made and be sure to include one's self in the list.

Step Nine. Made direct amends to such people wherever possible, except when to do so would injure them or others. Step 9 puts recovery into action. This is the opportunity to take a deep breath of the faith the alcoholic has in his or her Higher Power. Trusting in the system and in the process of letting go, the alcoholic faces the ones who have been hurt and offers amends. This is done with care for the other individual and for the self and no one should be put in danger in this endeavor.

The Maintenance Steps

Step 10. Continued to take personal inventory and when we were wrong promptly admitted it. The next three steps work together to maintain the recovery of the alcoholic. They lead to a spiritual awakening that comes slowly to some and quickly to others. Step 10 requires vigilance in the process of recovery. Humility again, comes into play. Being able to admit one's wrongs promptly saves a person from walking away with guilt, anger and resentment.

Step 11. Sought through prayer and meditation to improve our conscious contact with God, as we understood Him, praying only for knowledge of His will for us and the power to carry that out. Authentically working Step 11 maintains a connection with one's Higher Power. Asking for help, praying when one wakes up and lies down, giving thanks, meditating-these are all means by which the recovering alcoholic remains humble and relinquishes control to their Higher Power.

Step 12. Having had a spiritual awakening as the result of these Steps, we tried to carry this message to alcoholics and to practice these principles in all our affairs. In brief, this step is about passing the message on to others who need it, too. This is a spiritual practice because it intertwines one person to another. One individual's story becomes a part of the tapestry that blankets the recovery movement of Alcoholics Anonymous. As was mentioned in the introduction, Bill W. and Dr. Bob recognized the importance of sharing their experiences as a means by which to maintain their own recovery. This is a critical step in the AA legacy.

The Legacies

There are three legacies of Alcoholics Anonymous born out of the early years: Recovery, Unity and Service. The Legacies were handed over to the movement known as Alcoholics Anonymous on July 3, 1955 at the 20th Anniversary Convention in St. Louis, MO. This was a passing of the torch, so to speak. Those who had built this movement and allowed their recovery journey to be shared by so many-the old timers-passed on their gifts to the newest among them.

The first, the Legacy of Recovery, offers the lessons learned and the Steps to be taken to those who have yet experienced the spiritual journey of recovery and to those who may experience it anew. The Legacy of Unity ensures that the focus of Alcoholics Anonymous stays on recovering and sharing that recovery with others. The first of the Twelve Traditions says that "Our common welfare should come first; personal recovery depends upon A. A. unity" (Alcoholics Anonymous Comes of Age, p. 78). No one person is the face or the voice of A. A. Finally, the Legacy of Service is focused on sharing the message of recovery.

HOW TO HANDLE LYING ALCOHOLICS

When an alcoholic lies there's not much we can do about it. If we confront them they just continue lying about the situation. After attending a few support group meetings on dealing with problem drinkers, I finally realized that it was pointless to try and address the things the addict in my life was telling me that I knew were not true.

It took some real discipline on my part to NOT confront them about these secrets they were keeping from me. There was a purpose in not making a big deal about them not telling me the truth. The main objective was to stop fighting all of the time.

When an alcoholic is lying to us, we have a tendency to want to try to get them to tell us what really happened. When they continue to lie, we try even harder to get them to tell us the truth. This creates a never ending cycle of going around and around. We get frustrated and angry with them and have very little peace within.

Here's the key to breaking this habitual routine. Accept that lying is a part of what an alcoholic does. It is one of many character attributes that are common among problem drinkers. I know it's not really in our nature to just let someone get away with telling us lies, but this is the way to have more emotional peace within.

They are not going to change their behaviors. Therefore, the responsibility is on our shoulders to make changes to protect our own emotional well-being. When we can stop confronting them and just accept that lying is a big part of what they do, we will have more serenity in our lives. THEY ARE NOT GOING TO STOP LYING.

It's funny because I've written about this subject on one of my blogs about alcoholism. People write comments sometimes expressing their frustration with this type of situation. They seem to vent some of their anger toward me because they feel like I did not tell them how to get the alcoholic to tell them the truth. They get irritated when I tell them that the best way to cope with a lying alcoholic is to just be quiet and do not confront the lies.

Making changes in order to cope with a friend or loved one who has a drinking problem takes work on our part. The realization that we must make changes in how we respond to how they are living their lives is difficult to grasp.

When it comes to alcoholics lying, the reality of the situation is that they are "not" going to change. An alcoholic will continue to drink more than they reveal. They will not stop bending the truth of how they spent their time in a day either. They are living a world of denial and nothing that you or I do will change them. The best thing for our personal health is to accept that lying is what many alcoholics do and then quit confronting the lies.

It's funny because I've written about this subject on one of my blogs about alcoholism. People write comments sometimes expressing their frustration with this type of situation. They seem to vent some of their anger toward me because they feel like I did not tell them how to get the alcoholic to tell them the truth. They get irritated when I tell them that the best way to cope with a lying alcoholic is to just be quiet and do not confront the lies.

Making changes in order to cope with a friend or loved one who has a drinking problem takes work on our part. The realization that we must make changes in how we respond to how they are living their lives is difficult to grasp.

When it comes to alcoholics lying, the reality of the situation is that they are "not" going to change. An alcoholic will continue to drink more than they reveal. They will not stop bending the truth of how they spent their time in a day either. They are living a world of denial and nothing that you or I do will change them. The best thing for our personal health is to accept that lying is what many alcoholics do and then quit confronting the lies.

COPING WITH AN ALCOHOLIC WHO LIES CONSTANTLY

How can you tell when an alcoholic is lying? Their lips are moving. Coping with the lying nature of the problem drinker is better done through accepting the fact that lies are a way of life for most substance abusers.

Why do they lie so much? Let's face it; they are living in a world of denial. It's really not important to understand why they do this, just accept the fact and leave them alone when they twist the truth.

The sooner you can accept that lying is a part of the alcoholic's lifestyle the better you will be able to cope. Dealing with someone who is not telling the truth is frustrating because it causes us to want to argue with them that they are not telling the truth.

When we stop confronting them, then there will be a lot less finger pointing going on.

When we learn that we do not have to try and prove to them that we know they are telling us a lie, then our frustration level will go down. The truth of the matter is that their frustration level will go down as well. In return, all will be at peace in a dysfunctional kind of way. I can promise you that there will be a whole lot less arguing going on too.

What is the point of confronting an alcoholic who is lying anyway? You know they are just going to deny the truth and stand up for the false reality that they perceive to be truth.

Alcoholic liars come in every shape and form, from a teenage son, daughter, spouse, mom, dad, grandmother to a grandfather. When they are caught up in the grip of their addiction, they will have no respect for anyone, including themselves. If you can believe this, they really don't want to be they way that they are. It's an addiction that takes even the most respectable human beings into some of the shadiest places on earth.

The alcoholic lies about drinking because of the guilt and shame that accompanies their lifestyle. Have you ever know anyone who wanted to be an alcoholic when they grew up? Of course not; no one sets a goal to be addicted to some type of drug or substance.

The best way of coping (or, "dealing) with this problem is to just accept the truth and let them tell their lies without you pretending to be the private investigator who knows what really happened. Just let them live their dysfunctional life and you enjoy yours without the additional fight for the day. Unfortunately, lying is a comfortable way of life for the alcoholic. If you're going to cope with it, you must kick back and get comfortable with them not telling the truth as well.

HOW TO NOT BE AN ENABLER WITH AN ALCOHOLIC

When someone is able to help another person and has success in doing so, it make that person feel good about themselves that they were able to help someone in need.

There comes a time that you think are are helping someone, but in reality you are only hurting them. What I am referring to is helping a person with an addiction.

People with an alcohol addiction must be able to help themselves before someone else can help them. They need to want to be clean and sober. Once they have made their mind up that they do want a life of sobriety is when they should ask for outside help.

Through my experiences with alcohol addiction, people would talk to me about it and I would just listen, but I did not let any of what they said sink in. I really didn't care at all of what they said. I listened just to be polite to them.

An alcoholic must truly want to surrender to their addiction before anything will change in their lives. It may take a long time for that to happen, if it happens at all. With out determination, willingness or desire to become sober, the alcoholic will have possibly a very lonely life ahead of them if they are not willing to change.

Living with an alcoholic you can not be an enabler at all. You can not support them in any way, shape or form. They must figure out just how they will survive with out the help of others.

Families, spouses and friends tend to feel sorry for the addicted person, so they may lend or give money to them for their next bottle or six pack of beer. The alcoholic lies, makes up excuses, and tries anything to convince someone that this will be the last time I ask for money or any favors at all.

Allowing them to stay in the household after many long talks, with no success of them quitting drinking, also is not any help to them. They must make it on their own. When we allow them to just hang a round doing nothing but drink alcohol, they just figure they are on easy street and it's okay by us of how they are living. By saying nothing to them makes the alcoholic think we are giving permission towards their actions.

We must put our foot down making sure that the alcoholic knows what the consequences will be if they don't quit drinking and get the help they need.

The problem with saying such a thing to the alcoholic makes us feel very bad and certainly if the person is our spouse or child. They have to know you mean business and are serious about were they stand in your life.

THE BOTTOM LINE IS:

* Do not allow them to talk you into giving them money.

* Do not give them a choice of how they want to live their life in your home.

* Tell them they will live in your home under your conditions only.

* Stand up to them and don't let them walk all over you.

* Give them the opportunity to get the help they need.

* Encourage them that life will be so much better if they become sober.

* Tell them how much you love them and support them in their recovery.

* Tell them that you will stand by their side only when they decide to get help.

WHY ALCOHOLICS NEED SUPPORT

Alcohol consumption can relax one for while. Many people consume alcohol in order to escape tension and depression. With continuous alcohol consumption, the person gradually develops a tolerance and dependence on it. The long-term use of alcohol in large quantities can cause addiction. Alcoholics usually do not realise their growing problem and addiction to alcohol intake.

Alcohol consumption can have several negative consequences; alcoholics often find themselves in serious trouble due to their abnormal state of mind. Alcoholics usually do not admit their problems and also refuse to accept the reality. It might take several severe consequences for the alcoholic to realise how damaging alcohol is for him/her.

Even when an alcoholic realises his/her problem, he/she needs some time and support to take a step to correct the issue. The body of the alcoholic needs a specific amount of alcohol as it becomes dependent on it and craves for it. Alcoholics find it very hard to resist the temptation and face severe withdrawal symptoms as a result. Also if an alcoholic wants to quit, but his/her friends drink, then he/she cannot get rid of the habit.

Due to severe withdrawal symptoms the alcoholic faces extreme physical discomfort; therefore, quitting the habit on their own is very difficult. They need assistance and support to get over the problem. No one can force an alcoholic to leave the habit. Also the disease and addiction of alcohol makes the person lose hope and give up trying to quit the habit. The addiction makes the alcoholic lie, react violently, steal and do everything possible to drink alcohol. For an alcoholic, admitting the problem and talking to others about it is the most difficult thing to do, but it is also the first step for recovering.

Counselling is the major support needed by an alcoholic to prevent and treat the disease in time. The support that counselling provides help them know the reason as to why they drink and then find ways to treat the problem. Involvement of friends and family is the basis of family therapy which is a very important part of alcohol treatment.

Support of family and friends, helps an alcoholic live without alcohol. Alcoholics often try different ways to quit the drinking habit and if they do not have motivation, confidence, strength and encouragement, they go back to their drinking habit.

Fear that they would never get over the addiction to alcohol holds the alcoholics back. They feel very uncomfortable when dealing with the life changing decision to quit alcohol. It is very important to be supportive and helpful towards them.

Support plays a very important role in helping an alcoholic recover from the disease by letting him/her know that people do not judge or label them, they care for them. Support helps the alcoholic know that there is help available for them and they can deal with the problem. Support affects the behaviour of the alcoholic in indirect ways; therefore, it is very important.

HOW ALCOHOLISM
CONTROLS YOUR LIFE

It happens without warning. It creeps into your life and all of a sudden, you're hooked. At first you're the life of the party, and later you're the drunk of the party. When you're young, twenties and thirties, your body can handle all the booze, no problem. But mentally it impairs the way you view and feel the world around you.

Most of the time, alcoholics don't know that alcohol has taken hold of their life. This is called the denial stage. Alcoholics feel that if they can get up and go to work everyday, even though secretly they have an excruciating headache, they don't have a problem.

But what keeps the alcoholic going throughout the workday is in knowing that after work, they'll have those highballs or beers, which will in fact, make them feel like their old self again.

The problem is, that's not our old self, but our new old self on alcohol. You see, alcohol changes the person we are inside, not only does alcohol, with time, rot our insides, but it rots what comes from within us. What we do, how we treat others, and our spirituality.

The potential to be a whole person has been put on hold because of alcohol. The booze stunts the mental capacities and impairs the ability to see the world clearly enough to get passed the weakness and mistakes we make in life.

Alcohol is not only physically addicting, but mentally addicting as well. An alcoholic might believe they feel and look better while drinking; or they might THINK they can still drive a car; they don't realize their reflexes have slowed down; or they think they are better communicators after several martinis. But nothing is further from the truth.

Alcoholics don't know God. Ah yes, they say those things that your ears want to hear, and they even go to church every Saturday and Sunday, but what are their actions telling you. What fruits do you see shine bright in the alcoholic?

Spiritually speaking the alcoholic has allowed other sources to be His God, namely, Mr. Jim Beam. Until Mr. Beam gets out of the picture, he will literally master the alcoholic and his mind.

This is how alcohol takes control of the alcoholic's life!

Their thinking is literally impaired! The alcoholics don't really have a mind of their own. Alcohol speaks for them. Many decisions an alcoholic makes are based on or around drinking.

Most alcoholics think they are independent minded, but they are far from being independent thinkers. Unbeknownst to the alcoholic who is in denial is how dependent minded they really are. Always concerned about when and where they are going to get their next drink.

Alcoholics will make up acceptable reasons WHY they can drink. It's a fact of their life that seventy five percent of their waking minds are spent on thinking about drinking or drinking alcohol.

Alcoholics have a hard time growing up, even when they are adults. Their reasoning is not sound, but foolishness to the ears. Because they are locked in their own little world of alcohol, they never mature into the potential of who they can become because they are being drowned with alcoholic lies everyday.

What can the alcoholic do?

What can the enabler do?

It would be stupid for me to sit here and tell you to quit drinking; easier said than done right? Yep, if you're an alcoholic, I know what you're going through. What I can do though, is tell you what I did. If what I did sounds acceptable to you than give it a try.

First of all the enabler needs to get help by going to Alanon. Your getting help for your self will be helping the alcoholic in more ways than you'll ever know, believe me. In Alanon you will learn to not let the escapades of the alcoholic bother you. You will also learn to NOT rescue the alcoholic anymore! This aspect is so very important.

For the alcoholic, you need to read the New Testament everyday, even if you think it is boring and you don't want to read it, read it anyway. This is what I did. I got myself a pen and marked verses that sounded good even though I didn't actually understand it much. I dog-eared pages and my bible looked like something you would find on skid row. Thankfully this is not where I got my bible.

I really wanted to know more about God, and I would ask myself daily, "Who is God? What can God do for me?" I prayed a lot, I cried a lot, and I drink a lot.

I desperately wanted God to help me, but I didn't believe it. I was in denial that God could really help me. Many things go through your head when you are trying to discover truth and spirituality in your life when you are still drinking.

But one day several months later, still reading the bible and doing my own bible study and research, I decided how totally and completely disgusted I was with my self and my drinking, and I incessantly prayed for help from God.

"Consequently, faith comes from hearing the message, and the message is heard through the word of Jesus Christ." Romans 10:17

I asked God to take away the burden of Alcoholism from me and to take away the craving for alcohol as well. I told God that I finally trusted and believed in His power in my life, and to help me!

That was thirteen years ago, and I never had another drink, with the exception of a sip of punch at a wedding that was spiked and I didn't know it. I tasted it, and still, didn't want it or like it, I threw it out!

God will do what you ask of Him if you trust and believe in Him. He will take the heavy-laden burdens from your heart and mind; all you got to do is BELIEVE!

I didn't really know that much about "who God was" when I prayed for help on that day, thirteen years ago, but I didn't need to know the schematics of how God worked.

I needed to believe that God could and would take away my addiction for good. I needed to have faith enough to accept that for my life!

What God needed from me, was the knowing in my heart that I DID trust and believe in Him! Through my prayer, God read my heart and saved me.

In essence, it was my faith in God that saved me, nothing else.

How do you gain faith?

You gain faith by reading about the things God has done in the lives of others. By understanding how much God loves you and knowing He wants you to be all that He set out for you to be.

Basically, you just need to study the Bible daily, and you should never stop praying for what God wants for you in your life. Prayers aren't always going to get answered the way we would like, but let God take care of that part for you.

Don't stop praying silenting or reading the bible, God hears your pleas, and listens to your heart.

Some of you probably wonder what all this faith stuff is about since your prayers do not get met. But God does not work like this. His plan for us is not our plan for us.

And so understand, it is only when we already have faith in Him is when we stop praying selfishly, and ask God what He wants.

Two words can best describe faith, sure and certain. Having faith has two parts. The first part believes in God's character.

God is who He says He is!

The second part believes in His promise for us. He WILL do what He says!

When we believe that God will fulfill His promise for us without even seeing those promises materialize yet, we surely have true faith.

"Now faith is being sure of what we hope for and certain of what we do not see. This is what the ancients were commended for. By faith we understand that the universe was formed at God's command, so that what is seen was not made out of what was visible." Hebrews 11:1-3.

CHILDREN OF ALCOHOLIC PARENTS

Alcoholism is matter of serious concern, not confined to any group, culture or country. Universally it creates professional, social, financial, legal, medical, psychological, and familial problems. The cost of alcoholism to the society is staggering by any calculations. Lost working days, accidents and related disability, family disrupts and resulting juvenile problems, and direct medical complications of alcohol abuse add up to a significant proportion of loss to nations" economy and well being. Alcoholism thus becomes a complex phenomenon deserving attention from deferent angles.

Problem drinking within a family can lead to many types of stress and hard ships for family members. Increasing social isolation due to alcoholism is difficult for children to cope up. They behave increasingly withdrawn form peer group activities. Financial hardships become a factor and reductions are made to general standard of living. Physical hardships are seen either violence towards family members or in destruction of household things.

Family members especially spouse may be subjected to emotional deprivation and may perceive drinking as a form of rejection. This in turn causes the drinker to become increasingly preoccupied and plays a diminished role in family life and affairs.

Glassner and Loughlin (1987) emphasised on three aspects of parent-child relationships that are studied in alcoholics" families; basic care, consistency of expectations, and communications. Children find it difficult to cope with parental unpredictability or with unexplained withdrawal and sudden change in mood and temperament.

Children may suffer from physical and emotional neglect. Since all the family's energies are focused on the drinker, children are often neglected and their individual contributions go unacknowledged. This may result in acting out behavior, aggression, bedwetting, taunting, anxiety, withdrawal and isolation that in turn can increase the pressure on non-drinking parents. Another important problem is that children of alcoholics lack a satisfactory role model for their own behavior. Hence, the children represent an important high-risk group both because of their proneness to problem drinking during child hood and their proneness to problems in later life. Hence, the tragedy of alcoholism lies in its detrimental effects on future generation. Alcoholism of the individual affects not only the family but also even the basic fabric of the society. Alcohol causes poverty leading to crimes and prostitution that in turn ends up in the break down of any society's integrity and existence.

ALCOHOLISM - A DISEASE
OR A SYMPTOM

Alcohol is a drug that has been around for thousands of years. Ever since the discovery by Persian chemists around 600AD, has Alcohol been used for medicinal, recreational and industrial uses. Throughout years people have blended it, distilled it, mixed it, in order to make it more pallatable, and yet the affect on the body remains the same. It fundamentally changes the chemical balance within the body causes side effects. Some of these side effects are unwelcome, like slurred speech, imbalance, headaches. Some of the side effects have a more pleasing effect to others, like loosening inhibitions, more creativity and increased confidence. Alcohol, in excess, either over a long period, or serious excess in the short term, has serious side effects that can be irreversible. Major organ damage, resulting in medical treatment, transplants, or premature death, are the risks that someone who drinks to excess takes. So what is it?, that Alcohol gives the Alcoholic, that causes them to ignore the risk of death. That causes them to put others lives in their hands every time they get behind the wheel of a car. That bankrupts them, shattering their lives and others, and yet they still turn to it for the answer.

It is because of these chemical changes that an Alcoholic drinks. It is because of the change in thought pattern, or mood, or confidence, that an alcoholic continues to ignore, or deny, the potential life threatening risk they take every time they swallow the next mouthful. Deep down in the psyche of an Alcoholic, lies something that makes them unhappy. It is something that has been stored away in the "mental locker", festering and poisoning the character that is developing over the years. This can be an "event" that happened when younger, so traumatic that the memory is burnt within. A personal tragedy, or image, or abusive experience. When we are young, our emotions are developing as well as our physical bodies. Our mental capacity to cope with things is as inexperienced as our selves, and has yet to know how to react. So it stores it. It locks it away, so that it can be forgotten.

However, the damage has created a chain reaction in the character development. It has made the yet-to-be Alcoholic, less confident they they would have been, made them self-question their own worth, made them shy and passive rather than an assertive, self assured person. These feelings become the norm, and so are accepted as who we are. It is only later, after the discovery of Alcohol, that the door holding back the origin of the problem is unlocked. Unfortunately, Alcohol provides the key to this door, to just slightly open it. To release just a little of the memory. To just let the poison out slightly. Not enough for the Alcoholic to realise at first. Not quite enough for the Alcoholic to question what may be happening. The Alcoholic has found a solution to a problem they don't realise they have. The Alcoholic has discovered this magical liquid, that seems to make them feel better. The feelings of low self-esteem, that they have accepted, yet wished were treatable, are now vanished in a flash. The shy, quiet, passive person now magically transforms into a confident, assertive, jovial clown. This new behaviour seems so natural, and all it takes is a sip of this legal chemical. The effect itself is the drug. The addiction to the person, that deep down the Alcoholic has yearned to be, is what drives the Alcoholic to continue. Even if it means increasing the dose, which over time is inevitable. Even if it means denying other things in life, like food, sleep, intimacy, the power that the effect has created is the most important thing now. You never want to be that other person again, and you have found a way achieve that. Unfortunately it comes at a cost, and there is a big cost to pay.

Everyone, probably, has something about them that they would want to change. For some its outside features, like liposuction, or enhancements, and because these are external, they are more obvious to the individual. For others, though, they wish they could change their character. Mental changes are far more invisible. They want more confidence, or more assertiveness, or be funnier. There are solutions to this also, that do not come in a Litre Bottle.

There are techniques to boost confidence that don't involve Vodka, or Gin, and although they take longer, and more work, they have the

346

same effect. With help the effects can get to the root cause. They can nullify the poison, that has been polluting the character. The person that emerges happy, healthy, and looking forward to life. The next time you take a drink, be truthful to yourself, and ask yourself why. The answer to this, and the consequences you take based on the answer, could just save you from suffering.

LIVING WITH AN ALCOHOLIC

It really doesn't matter if we're the child, spouse or parent of an alcoholic; the abuse, pain, self-doubt and fear are severe and frequent. We spend a lot of compassionate effort trying to help alcoholics recover, but very little on the loved ones, some of whom may be scarred for life. If you have a loved one who is an alcoholic, this chapter is for you. If you're addicted to alcohol and have loved ones trying to help you, please consider this article a wake-up call.

Secrets And Lies: Alcohol addicts need to be woken up because the biggest lie they tell is to themselves, "I don't have a problem." As much as you love the alcoholic in your family, that lie is what makes it easy to lie to you. My father would say he'll be at my game, my play, my graduation...usually lies. When he didn't arrive, it was always because he was tired. Funny how tired you can get after a few drinks...or before a few. He did the best he could, given his addictions, so, I'm not whining...Just letting you know I know what you're going through. Some alcoholics claim to not drink and have hours of secret time away from home, all with convenient lies to hide what's really happening. Of course, the truth can't help but be revealed when they overindulge and stumble into the house, get in an accident or get arrested. Sadly, most of the time, these incidents are only followed by more lies, this time about quitting or cutting back. Funny, how easy it is to believe the lies just one more time.

Coping-Not Codependence: One of the sad things about being codependent to an alcoholic is how easy it is to believe their lies. Our love for them overshadows the obvious truth...and we begin to live in denial just like the one we love. We become addicted to the neediness of our alcoholic loved one. Instead, we need to learn to cope with them rather than enable them. No, we won't believe their words...only their actions. We will protect the rest of the family from them but we won't enable them by excusing or supporting them in any way as long as they continue in their addiction. Coping with an alcoholic means being tough and confronting them. It means setting clear boundaries and not changing them just because the addict makes a fuss. It means letting them live in the consequences of their actions...even if they lose their job or freedom due to a jail sentence. Calling in to work, making excuses, bailing them out of jail actually helps them continue in their addiction. You don't love an alcoholic by holding them up. Loving them means letting them hit the ground until they learn to hate falling more than they love drinking.

The Only Love Of An Addict: When we give in to the manipulation and the alcoholic rewards us with words of admiration and love, it's just another lie. The words seem sincere because they are spoken to you, but the words of love about the bottle, and no one else. Alcoholics hate themselves and are incapable of loving anyone...not their kids, their spouse, their parents...they are all pawns to be used to get that next drink. Drinking isn't an alcoholic's first love, it's the only love. Until that bond is broken, no one else will be allowed in.

Recovery Or Rejection: This article may seem as though I think it impossible for an alcoholic to recover. It may surprise you to know I'm a recovered alcoholic. I didn't get to recovery because people excused me. It was only after I realized I had become my Dad, with his drunkenness, violence and lies...only when I saw that I would get this addiction under control or lose my wife, my career and everything. That was bottom for me...what brought me to find help and get this addiction behind me. I was lucky and I had help from God and others around me...not help to get drunk, but help to live sober.

Unfortunately, if nothing else works for your alcoholic, sometimes they need to know there are only two choices...begin recovery or be rejected. A drug addict I knew was squatting in an abandoned house with her 3 small children and her supplier boyfriend, with no furniture, piles of uncontained trash and food scraps next to the uncovered mattresses and piles of unwashed, filthy clothes. I can't begin to describe the smell. She had to have her three children taken away from her before she would enter rehab and get clean. The last time I saw her, she was healthy, well-dressed, employed and had her children back with her. The greatest act of love toward this woman came from a government agency by taking her children.

If your alcoholic won't quit, as hard as it is, the greatest act of love you can offer is to withhold your support, your help, yourself and your love from them. This is their best chance for recovery. If the addict won't quit even then, the choice was made by the addict...and by you. This was your last and greatest act of love...to give them up in hopes they would give up the bottle.

Living With An Alcoholic is never easy, coping with secrets and lies and being manipulated for that next drink. If the bottle turns out to be their one true love, often, the only option is to leave them and salvage your life. Hopefully, with your firm boundaries, a little luck and a lot of God's help, your alcoholic will give it up and live in recovery, proving you're their one true love and eventually learning to love even themselves.

FACTS ABOUT ALCOHOLICS AND ALCOHOLISM

There is a lot of information available on the web for, and about, alcoholics. Titles of articles range from "Alcoholism and Alcohol Addiction" to "Zen Meditation in Treating Alcoholism". Though these articles are all helpful in their own way few of them seem willing to speak the frank and candid truth about active alcoholics. This article outlines the simple truths about people who drink too much, too often and to excess.

1. All Alcoholics are Liars

There isn't one actively drinking alcoholic in the world who isn't a liar. They lie to themselves about their drinking and they lie to everyone else about everything. You can't accept one thing that comes out of their mouth as the truth. They come home late and say they were working late. They have seven drinks and say they had three. They tell you they got a promotion at work and they got fired. They say they are looking for work and they aren't. Their lies twist and deceive and make the people around them doubt their own reality. Their lies are poison to relationships, friendships and work colleagues.

2. All Alcoholics Are Manipulators

Alcoholics use people to meet their own ends. They make people angry and in the process prove to themselves that people are cruel to them. They convince their lives to ring up the workplace and tell the boss they are sick. The make promises to their children and don't keep them, then manage to make the children feel bad for putting their parent under pressure. Their manipulations extend to every part of their lives. They will pitch one person against another, telling stories to their parents to make them believe that a brother or sister is against them. They manipulate every event in life to their own advantage and in so doing cause people to never know who they can trust.

3. All Alcoholics Are In Love with Drink

Nothing has more sex appeal to the alcoholic than drink. Drink is the scantily clad woman becoming them from a window or the half dressed stud lifting weights in the gym. People are objects to the alcoholic, objects to be used as a reason to drink. If someone praises the alcoholic it becomes either a reason to rejoice in drink or bury the reality they do not deserve praise in drink. It they get a raise or job promotion it is a reason to drink; if they lose a job it is a reason to drink. If they see someone they fancy they need a drink in order to approach them. If they are rejected they drink to drown the sting. Their wives and husbands exist to them only as a way to get to a drink. Their children are a reason to drink. Sport is a reason to drink. Family celebrations are a reason to drink. Holidays are a reason to drink. Everything in the life of an alcoholic is used as a means of getting to their one true love-drink.

4. All Alcoholics Know the Truth about Themselves

Alcoholics know their behaviour is reprehensible, that they are liars and manipulators. In order to protect themselves from the terrible truth they create a false front of superiority and put others down as a means to look good. The alcoholic husband will tell their wife they are the reason there is food on the table. The alcoholic wife will tell her husband if it weren't for her he wouldn't have a social life. This inflated sense of self-esteem, which masks their inner sense of worthlessness. Hiding this horrible truth from others necessitates making others feel inferior, foolish and stupid on a regular basis.

5. There is No Such Things as a Functional Alcoholic

They myth of the functional alcoholic is deeply embedded in society. So many people addicted to alcohol believe that if they go to work, do a day's work, contribute to the family income and show up at important family events they are functional. The truth is they are not functional in any sense at all. The vast majority of them, men and women alike, are emotionally regressed, socially inhibited, psychological cripples individuals. They are unable to function without their daily fix of alcohol, unable to do a days work with the reward of a good drinking session at its end and unable to express any sincere emotion to those closest to them.

ALCOHOLISM AND ITS ABUSE

With many different opinions and approaches it is not easy to give a definition of alcoholism. Definitions in general often evoke contrasting views which can be rather confusing. In America alcoholism is accepted as a disease, whereas in Europe generally, it is not seen as a medical problem, and therefore hardly any funds are made available to find a 'medical solution'.

The definition of alcoholism remains vague but overall we can say that alcoholism is a form of problem drinking and involves a physical dependence on alcoholic drinks.

But what about the people affected by it? Are they interested in a fancy definition? Probably not. Partners, family members and friends of alcoholics are trying to make sense of a life out of control, a life of lies. People are trying to make ends meet and there is desperation and often violence, both verbally and physically. They don't care about fancy studies and conclusions and are more interested in advice on living with an alcoholic and how to help an alcoholic.

The alcoholic, held hostage by the alcohol, feels alone and in deep conflict with those around him and deep down inside, also with him or herself. They probably know the problems alcohol abuse can cause. They probably know what it must mean to their loved ones to live with an alcoholic, but they feel there is no choice, that there is no way out. Only escape through the numbing effect of alcohol to cover possible feelings of guilt and the apparent easy solution of denial. Alcoholism and its definition are irrelevant and empty terms.

Alcoholism isn't even defined by the amount a person drinks, but by the effect drinking has on any area of someone's life, such as:

• Arguments with family and friends about how much someone should drink

• Lying or hiding your drinking habits

• Needing a drink so you can relax

• Not remembering what you did during a drinking session (black out)

• Rather spending money on alcohol than on food

• Drinking to feel better about yourself

• Drinking more than you intended to on a regular basis

• Drinking while you know it can be physically dangerous, like drinking and driving

• Neglecting your responsibilities at home and/or at work

• Using alcohol as a self-medication for other health problems, such as anxiety, depression, etc.

• Relying on alcohol to function

• Feel physically compelled to have a drink, for example shaking.

It is not the easiest of tasks to be able to differentiate when the drinking pattern changes from moderate and social to kind of a problem drinking. The worst part about the total process is that when you are trying to dig up alcohol due to some problems that you are facing, it has to be understood that the situation is grave. Alcoholics slowly start losing their grip of understanding and presence of mind making them susceptible to the process of abuse leading the alcohol and its effects to gate-crash into the character of the person concerned. Understanding the problem is a big step towards solving it and in this scenario, to be able to recognise the line of border between alcohol and the abuse that comes with it is a major area of concern.

Features and Signs of Alcoholism and Alcohol Abuse:

• Know Yourself: It is really important to understand at the very first step that you have a drinking problem or not. This can happen if you are lying to others about drinking, feeling guilty about the fact that you drink or drink more than intended to. These are the basic questions a person needs to ask himself to ascertain the current situation that he/she is in and if the results for these queries are correct, steps have to be taken sooner than never.

• Neglecting Responsibilities: With the continuous outburst of your brain for the need of alcohol in your body due to sensitisation, the only priority that reaches is to take care of your alcohol routine. Thereby, you slowly start neglecting your responsibilities and prioritise drinking.

• Lack of Tolerance: With a continuous routine for drinking, the body's ability to tolerate situations without alcohol get lost to a great extent. Signs such as anxiety, sweating, headache, fatigue, depression, loss of appetite and insomnia may arise, causing serious levels of health problems.

• Denial and lying: This is one of the moments when you start lying about drinking and denying it, making you to feel guilty about it.

So is there a solution?

Definitely, yes! Everyday tons of alcoholics suffering from its abuse are undergoing treatment using:

• Alcohol treatment centres

• Alcohol rehabs

• Process of alcohol detoxification

The thing that needs to be understood is that the problem lies within oneself and if someone can take that alcohol frenzy character out of the mind and if the alcohol withdrawal symptoms are understood initially, the battle is won!

CONCLUSION

Most people love their families and spouses regardless of hardship and suffering they may experience. People are connected to their loved ones. If your loved one is lying, stealing and hurting themselves or you because of drug or alcohol abuse, do the rules change?

Drug and alcohol abusers forget quickly. Promises and agreements are forgotten.

What are the right ways to rescue a drug addict or alcoholic? Most families believe they are doing the right thing, but are surprised or shocked when a drug or alcohol abusing loved one doesn't respond the way they wanted to.

I hear the same big mistakes being committed by families while trying to save their drug / alcohol abusing loved one. How does one provide a space for addicts to recover without helping them to continue their abusing lifestyle?

If you have a loved one abusing drugs and alcohol and don't know why they continue to abuse despite promising they'll stop, you may be making one or more of these major mistakes.

CPSIA information can be obtained
at www.ICGtesting.com
Printed in the USA
BVHW041649300421
606221BV00010B/1239

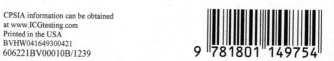

9 781801 149754